MEDICAL TOURISM : CODES AND GUIDELINES

MEDICAL TOURISM : CODES AND GUIDELINES

G.R. Chatak

CYBER TECH PUBLICATIONS
4264/3, Ansari Road, Daryaganj, New Delhi-110002 (India)
Ph.: 011-23244078, 011-43559448 Fax: 011-23280028
E-Mail: cyberpublicationsdelhi@yahoo.com
Website: www.cybertechpublications.com

MEDICAL TOURISM : CODES AND GUIDELINES

G.R. Chatak

First Edition 2010

Asian Offset Printers

Published by :

G.S. Rawat for **Cyber Tech Publications**
4264/3, Ansari Road, Daryaganj, New Delhi-110002 (India)
Ph.: 011-23244078, 011-43559448 Fax: 011-23280028
E-Mail: cyberpublicationsdelhi@yahoo.com
Website: www.cybertechpublications.com

Preface

Medical tourism is the practice of a patient "outsourcing" healthcare services to an area outside of his/her home country. Medical travel is becoming more popular, as more people realize its benefits. The main benefits of health tourism include getting the opportunity to travel to an exotic destination and reaping potentially big monetary savings. Many common operations overseas cost a fraction of what they might cost in the United States. For instance, the average cost of rhinoplasty (or nose job) in the U.S. is $6,000; the same procedure in Costa Rica costs only $1,500. The savings of $4,500 is more than enough to cover your travel expenses, and you'll get to travel to a new destination. Medical Tourism Guide.org is committed to bringing you the very best information regarding the advantages and disadvantages of medical travel, or health tourism.

Medical tourism also affords the chance to get in a little sightseeing before or after your treatment. You can spend your recovery relaxing under an umbrella on a scenic beach or a mountain resort or even just enjoying the benefits of a high class hotel's room service. In some places, medical tourism packages may be all inclusive, providing you with medical staff on call at your lodgings. All these benefits don't come risk-free, however, but a majority of the risk associated with medical tourism can be managed with careful planning and research. There are a number of options available to those seeking treatment outside their home country and this website as well as others can be a great resource to figuring out which destination is best for you. Popular destinations include Brazil, Costa Rica, India, Malaysia, South Africa, and Turkey, just to name a few.

— *Author*

CONTENTS

1
Introduction

Medical tourism (also called medical travel, health tourism or global healthcare) is a term initially coined by travel agencies and the mass media to describe the rapidly-growing practice of traveling across international borders to obtain health care. Such services typically include elective procedures as well as complex specialized surgeries such as joint replacement (knee/hip), cardiac surgery, dental surgery, and cosmetic surgeries. As a practical matter, providers and customers commonly use informal channels of communication-connection-contract, and in such cases this tends to mean less regulatory or legal oversight to assure quality and less formal recourse to reimbursement or redress, if needed.

Leisure aspects typically associated with travel and tourism may be included on such medical travel trips. Prospective medical tourism patients need to keep in mind the extra cost of travel and accommodations when deciding on treatment locations. A specialized subset of medical tourism is reproductive tourism, which is the practice of traveling abroad to undergo in-vitro fertilization and other assisted reproductive technology treatments.

The concept of medical tourism is not a new one. The first recorded instance of medical tourism dates back thousands of years to when Greek pilgrims traveled from all over the Mediterranean to the small territory in the Saronic Gulf called Epidauria. This territory was the sanctuary of the healing god Asklepios. Epidauria became the original travel destination for medical tourism. Spa towns and sanitariums may be considered an early form of medical tourism. In eighteenth century England, for example, medtrotters visited spas because they were places with supposedly health-giving mineral waters, treating diseases from gout to liver disorders and bronchitis.

DESCRIPTION

Factors that have led to the increasing popularity of medical travel include the high cost of health care, long wait times for certain procedures, the ease and affordability of international travel, and improvements in both technology and standards of care in many countries. Medical tourists can come from anywhere in the world, including Europe, the UK, Middle East, Japan, the United States, and Canada. This is because of their large populations, comparatively high wealth, the high expense of health care or lack of health care options locally, and increasingly high expectations of their populations with respect to health care.

A large draw to medical travel is convenience and speed. Countries that operate public health-care systems are often so taxed that it can take considerable time to get non-urgent medical care. The time spent waiting for a procedure such as a hip replacement can be a year or more in Britain and Canada; however, in Costa Rica, Singapore, Hong Kong, Thailand, Cuba, Colombia, Philippines or India, a patient could feasibly have an operation the day after their arrival. In Canada, the number of procedures in 2005 for which people were waiting was 782,936.

Additionally, patients are finding that insurance either does not cover orthopedic surgery (such as knee/hip replacement) or imposes unreasonable restrictions on the choice of the facility, surgeon, or prosthetics to be used. Medical tourism for knee/hip replacements has emerged as one of the more widely accepted procedures because of the lower cost and minimal difficulties associated with the traveling to/from the surgery. Colombia provides a knee replacement for about $5,000 USD, including all associated fees, such as FDA- approved prosthetics and hospital stay-over expenses. However, many clinics quote prices that are not all inclusive and include only the surgeon fees associated with the procedure. According to an article by the University of Delaware publication, UDaily:

> *"The cost of surgery in India, Thailand or South Africa can be one-tenth of what it is in the United States or Western Europe, and sometimes even less. A heart-valve replacement that would cost $200,000 or more in the US, for example, goes for $10,000 in India--and that includes round-trip airfare and a brief vacation package. Similarly, a metal-free dental bridge worth $5,500 in the US costs $500 in India, a knee replacement in Thailand with six days of physical therapy costs about one-fifth of what it would in the States, and Lasik eye surgery worth $3,700 in the US is available in many other countries for only $730. Cosmetic surgery savings are even greater: A full facelift that would cost $20,000 in the US runs about $1,250 in South Africa."*

Popular medical travel worldwide destinations include: India, Brunei, Cuba, Colombia, Costa Rica, Hong Kong, Hungary, Jordan, Lithuania, Malaysia, The Philippines, Singapore, South Africa, Thailand, and recently, Saudi Arabia, UAE, Tunisia and New Zealand. Popular cosmetic surgery travel destinations include: Argentina, Bolivia, Brazil, Colombia, Costa Rica, Cuba, Mexico and Turkey. In South America, countries such as Argentina, Bolivia, Brazil and Colombia lead on plastic surgery medical skills relying on their experienced plastic surgeons.

It is estimated that 1 in 30 Argentineans have had plastic surgery procedures, making this population the most operated in the world after the US and Mexico. In Bolivia and Colombia, plastic surgery has also become quite common. According to the "Sociedad Boliviana de Cirugia Plastica y Reconstructiva", more than 70% of middle and upper class women in the country have had some form of plastic surgery. Colombia also provides advanced care in cardiovascular and transplant surgery.

In Europe Belgium, Poland and Slovakia are also breaking into the business. South Africa is taking the term "medical tourism" very literally by promoting their "medical safaris". However, perceptions of medical tourism are not always positive.

In places like the US, which has high standards of quality, medical tourism is viewed as risky. Nonetheless, the number of Americans who are going abroad for health care is increasing. In some parts of the world, wider political issues can influence where medical tourists will choose to seek out health care.

Health tourism providers have developed as intermediaries to unite potential medical tourists with provider hospitals and other organisations. Companies are beginning to offer global health care options that will enable North American and European patients to access world health care at a fraction of the cost of domestic care. Companies that focus on medical value travel typically provide nurse case managers to assist patients with pre- and post-travel medical issues. They also help provide resources for follow-up care upon the patient's return.

INTERNATIONAL HEALTHCARE ACCREDITATION

Because standards are important when it comes to health care, there are parallel issues around medical tourism, international healthcare accreditation, evidence-based medicine and quality assurance.

In the United States, Joint Commission International (JCI) fulfills an accreditation role, while in the UK and Hong Kong, the Trent International Accreditation Scheme is a key player. The different international healthcare accreditation schemes vary in quality, size, cost, intent and the skill of their marketing. They also vary in terms of cost to hospitals and healthcare institutions using them.

Many international hospitals today see obtaining JCI accreditation as a way to attract American patients and the number of JCI-accredited facilities has increased significantly over the last several years. Increasingly, some hospitals are looking towards dual international accreditation, perhaps having both JCI to cover potential US clientele and Trent for potential British and European clientele. Other relevant organizations include:

- The Society for International Healthcare Accreditation (SOFIHA), a free-to-join group providing a forum for discussion and for the sharing of ideas and good practice by providers of international healthcare accreditation and users of the same. The primary role of this organisation is to promote a safe hospital environment for patients.
- HealthCare Tourism International, the first US-based non-profit to accredit the non-clinical aspects of health tourism, such as language issues, business practices, and false or misleading advertising prevention. The group provides accreditation for all major groups involved in the health tourism industry including hotels, recovery facilities, and medical tourism booking agencies.

RISKS

Medical tourism carries some risks that locally-provided medical care does not. Some countries, such as India, Malaysia, Costa Rica, or Thailand have very different infectious disease-related epidemiology to Europe and North America. Exposure to diseases without having built up natural immunity can be a hazard for weakened individuals, specifically with respect to gastrointestinal diseases (e.g Hepatitis A, amoebic dysentery, paratyphoid) which could weaken progress, mosquito-transmitted diseases, influenza, and tuberculosis (e.g., 75% of South Africans have latent TB). However, because in poor tropical nations diseases run the gamut, doctors seem to be more open to the possibility of considering any infectious disease, including HIV, TB, and typhoid, while there are cases in the West where patients were consistently misdiagnosed for years because such diseases are perceived to be "rare" in the West.

The quality of post-operative care can also vary dramatically, depending on the hospital and country, and may be different from US or European standards. Also, travelling long distances soon after surgery can increase the risk of complications. Long flights can be bad for those with heart (thrombosis) or breathing-related problems. Other vacation activities can be problematic as well - for example, scars may become darker and more noticeable if they sunburn while healing. To minimise these problems, medical tourism patients often combine their medical trips with vacation time set aside for rest and recovery in the destination country. Also, health facilities treating medical tourists may lack an adequate complaints policy to deal appropriately and fairly with complaints made by dissatisfied patients.

LEGAL ISSUES

By traveling outside their home country for medical care, medical tourists may encounter unfamiliar ethical and legal issues. The limited nature of litigation in non-US countries is one reason for the lower cost of care overseas. While some countries currently presenting themselves as attractive medical tourism destinations provide some form of legal remedies for medical malpractice, these legal avenues may be unappealing to the medical tourist.

Should problems arise, patients might not be covered by adequate personal insurance or might be unable to seek compensation via malpractice lawsuits.

Hospitals and/or doctors in some countries may be unable to pay the financial damages awarded by a court to a patient who has sued them, owing to the hospital and/or the doctor not possessing appropriate insurance cover and/or medical indemnity. However new insurance products are available that protect the patient should an alleged medical malpractice occur overseas.

ETHICAL ISSUES

There can be major ethical issues around medical tourism. For example, the illegal purchase of organs and tissues for transplantation has been alleged in countries such as India and China. Medical tourism may raise broader ethical issues for the countries in which it is promoted. For example in India, some argue that a "policy of 'medical tourism for the classes and health missions for the masses' will lead to a deepening of the inequities" already embedded in the health care system.

EMPLOYER-SPONSORED HEALTH CARE

A few US employers have started offering incentives in their employee benefit packages such as paying for air travel and waiving out-of-pocket expenses for care outside of the US. For example, in January 2008, Hannaford Bros., a supermarket chain based in Maine, began paying the entire medical bill for employees to travel to Singapore for hip and knee replacements, including travel for the patient and companion. Other employers have been less public about their benefit changes.

Medical travel packages can integrate with all types of health insurance, including limited benefit plans, preferred provider organizations and high deductible health plans. Insurers are beginning to establish partnerships with overseas health providers to treat their insureds. The article cites a BlueCross BlueShield of South Carolina representative who had a colonoscopy at Bumrungrad International Medical Center in Bangkok.

According to a recent case study interview in The Health Care Globalization Report, a major employee benefits management company, Plan Benefit Services, accompanied a group of employers to Bangkok and Singapore to visit facilities. This is seen as significant since up to this point, most visitors to foreign hospitals were patients, health plans and medical travel companies. According to the report, the employers attending were very close to making benefit changes that would incentivize employees to seek care overseas. In another publication, Fast Company Magazine, a much lengthier story discusses the globalization of healthcare and how an employee benefits decision-maker for the City of Myrtle Beach fully supports overseas care, having been a patient himself for a colonoscopy.

DESTINATIONS

Asia/Pacific

China

Although not necessarily considered a destination for such procedures as cancer treatment, hip replacement or treatment for heart disease; China is becoming a destination for Westerners who want to take advantage of stem cell treatments that are still considered experimental or have yet to be approved in their home country for conditions such as paralysis.

Hong Kong

Hong Kong has 12 private hospitals and 39 public hospitals in 2006, providing 3124 and 27755 beds respectively. A wide range of health care services are offered. All 12 of Hong Kong's private hospitals have been surveyed and accredited by the UK's Trent Accreditation Scheme since early 2001. This has been a major factor in the ascent of standards in Hong Kong's private hospitals.

The Trent scheme works closely with the hospitals it assesses to generate standards appropriate to the locality (with respect to culture, geography, public health, primary care interfaces etc.), and always uses combinations of UK-sourced and Hong Kong-sourced surveyors. Some of Hong Kong's private hospitals have now gone on to obtain dual international accreditation, with both Trent and JCI (and have therefore attained a standard surpassing some of the best hospitals in Thailand and Singapore). Others are looking towards dual international accreditation with Trent and the Australian group. Hong Kong public hospitals have yet to commit to external accreditation.

India

India is known in particular for heart surgery, hip resurfacing and other areas of advanced medicine. The government and private hospital groups are committed to the goal of making India a leader in the industry. The industry's main appeal is low-cost treatment. Most estimates claim treatment costs in India start at around a tenth of the price of comparable treatment in America or Britain. India is becoming the destination of choice for US citizens seeking complicated, high-end medical procedures. Estimates of the value of medical tourism to India go as high as $2 billion a year by 2012. The Indian government is taking steps to address infrastructure issues that hinder the country's growth in medical tourism.

The south Indian city of Chennai has been declared India's Health Capital, as it nets in 45% of health tourists from abroad and 30-40% of domestic health tourists. Dental care has also caught on in India, with tourists coupling stays in cities like Udaipur with general check-ups and complex procedures.

Israel

Israel is emerging as a popular destination for medical tourists. Its modern, field-leading set of physicians and medical facilities are often used by international patients. In 2006, 15,000 foreigners travelled to the country for medical procedures, bringing in $40 million of revenue. Medical tourists choose Israel for several reasons. Some come from European nations such as Bulgaria where certain procedures are not available. Others come to Israel, perhaps most commonly from the US, because they can receive quality health care at a fraction of the cost it would be at home, for both surgeries and in-vitro fertilization treatments. Other medical tourists come to Israel to visit the Dead Sea, a world-famous therapeutic resort. The Israel Ministry of Tourism and several professional medical services providers have set out to generate awareness of Israel's medical capabilities.

Malaysia

Malaysia has ambitions to develop itself as a medical tourism hub. The country has excellent hospitals, English is widely spoken, and many staff have been trained to a high level in the UK or in the US. There is a highly active Association for Private Hospitals of Malaysia working to develop medical tourism. While Malaysia has a national accreditation scheme (MSQH), few of Malaysia's hospitals currently hold international healthcare accreditation, whether British, American or Australian.

New Zealand

New Zealand is a relatively new player to the medical travel market, focusing on non-acute surgical procedures and fertility treatment. Like other Commonwealth countries, New Zealand's medical system is based on the British health system. Most of its specialist physicians have received training in New

Zealand and the US or the UK, and all use English as their first language. The costs of private healthcare are significantly cheaper than the US or the UK, with packages (airfare, accommodation, medical service etc) for procedures like hip replacement, or coronary artery bypass costing in total approximately 40% of the procedure cost alone in the US. Many private hospitals in New Zealand are accredited by the national accreditation agency Quality Health New Zealand (QHNZ). QHNZ, like JCI, is a member of the International Society for Quality in healthcare or ISQua.

Philippines

The Philippines has been growing as a destination for medical tourism. Procedures can be performed at a fraction of the amount that a patient would spend on the same procedure in the US or Europe. Philippine medical and nursing curricula are more challenging than in many in Southeast Asia, and many Filipino doctors have acquired their postgraduate or fellowship training from well-known institutions in the US, the UK and other developed countries.

Medical centers in Metro Manila have complied to ISO standards, and are periodically and regularly undergo accreditations from Philippine's Department of Health. Others have already accredited by the American accreditation group Joint Commission International (JCI), while some have appied to join the UK-sourced Trent Accreditation Scheme.

Singapore

In 2006, some 410,000 visitors came to Singapore for health care services ranging from basic screening and cosmetic surgery to high-end surgical procedures and complex speciality care in areas such as cardiology, neurology, obstetrics and gynecology, oncology, ophthalmology, orthopedics and pediatrics among others. With internationally-accredited hospitals and speciality centres, a global reputation as a medical convention and training centre, and a fast-growing basic and clinical research hub, Singapore has established itself as a leading medical destination, serving medical travellers from around the world. In 2003, the Political and Economic Risk Consultancy (PERC) ranked

Singapore's health care system as the third best in the world and the country best prepared to deal with a major medical crisis in Asia. The World Health Organization ranked Singapore's health care system as the best in Asia and sixth best in the world in 2000.

Many patients come from neighboring countries, such as Indonesia and Malaysia, and patient numbers from Indochina, South Asia, the Middle East and Greater China are growing. Patients from developed countries such as the United States and the UK are also beginning to choose Singapore as their medical travel destination for relatively affordable health care services in a clean cosmopolitan city. However, Singapore hospitals have opted to stick exclusively with American-sourced JCI accreditation rather than look at hospital accreditation from the UK or Australia,. Singapore doctors tend to make use of UK sourced postgraduate qualifications, such as MRCP and MRCS, to indicate high quality, and most Singapore doctors are members of the British-based Medical Protection Society. "SingaporeMedicine" is a multi-agency government-industry partnership committed to strengthening Singapore's position as Asia's leading medical hub and promoting Singapore as a world-class destination for advanced patient care.

Thailand

Medical tourism is a growing segment of Thailand's tourism and health-care sectors. In 2005, one Bangkok hospital took in 150,000 treatment seekers from abroad. In 2006, medical tourism was projected to earn the country 36.4 billion baht. Thailand offers everything from cardiac surgery to organ transplants at a price much lower than the US or Europe. Thai medicine also features a higher, more personalized level of nursing care than westerners are accustomed to receiving in hospitals at home. One patient who received a coronary artery bypass surgery at Bumrungrad International hospital in Bangkok said the operation cost him US$12,000 (8,200 euros), as opposed to the $100,000 (68,000 euros) he estimated the operation would have cost him at home.

Hospitals in Thailand are a popular destination for other Asians. Another hospital that caters to medical tourists, Bangkok

Hospital, has a Japanese wing and Phyathai Hospitals Group has interpreters for over 22 languages, besides the English-speaking medical staff. When Nepal Prime Minister Girija Prasad Koirala needed medical care in 2006, he went to Bangkok. Today many Thai physicians hold US or UK professional certification. Several Thai hospitals have relationships with educational facilities in the US and UK (for example, Sheffield Hallam University has links with Bangkok}. One Thai hospital, Bumrungrad International, states that many of its doctors and staff are trained in the UK, Europe and the US. Bumrungrad International was accredited most recently in 2005 by an American group in order to ensure an international standard of medical services.

The US consular information sheet gives the Thai health care system high marks for quality, particularly facilities in Bangkok, although the World Health Organization ranks the Thai healthcare system at number 47, which is below the USA's ranking at 37 and the United Kingdom's ranking at 18. The UK's Foreign and Commonwealth Office web site states "There are excellent international hospitals in Bangkok but they can be expensive".

Europe

Cyprus

Cyprus has a strong medical heritage and possesses a high-quality healthcare system modeled on the British system, and the country has a number of private hospitals which are seeking to develop medical tourism. Many of the best hospitals have medical staff trained in the UK, Germany and other leading European countries. As of yet, many Cypriot hospitals have not sought international healthcare accreditation.

Germany

Germany has long been a medical tourism destination for people from the Middle East and North Africa. Now with a reduction in tension between East and West, many Russians and other Eastern Europeans are seeking treatment in Germany. British and Canadians, no longer willing to wait for treatment in their home country, are also traveling to Germany for treatment. Americans are also heading to Germany for the latest in spine surgery and novel cancer treatments and much lower prices than they would pay in the US. However, few German hospitals as yet have international healthcare accreditation.

Malta

Malta has a strong medical heritage and possesses a high-quality healthcare system modeled on the British system. The population is English-speaking. Malta is part of the European Union, a member of the Commonwealth of Nations, and has the euro as its currency. There are a number of private hospitals within Malta which are developing medical tourism, especially for UK residents. Some Maltese hospitals have applied to join the Trent Accreditation Scheme from the United Kingdom.

Portugal

Portugal's health care system is highly rated by the World Health Organization's ranking of the world's health systems, rated 12th of 191 countries. This is a European Union country with regulatory bodies that certify doctors and health facilities, thereby protecting patients' rights. Proximity to the US and Northern Europe reduce patients' travel risks, while Portugal's mild climate is well-suited for convalescence. English is widely spoken by the majority of the population and Portugal is well known for its low crime rate. Dental clinics and cosmetic surgery facilities are popular. Prices are low when compared with similar procedures performed in the UK or the US. Other medical procedures include bariatrics, orthopedics, cardiology and eye surgery.

Spain

Spain's strong economy over recent years have provided for modern hospitals and well-trained health care professionals, making it an up-and-coming medical tourism destination.

Turkey

Turkey has attracted medical tourists from Europe and is seeking to build on its geothermal resources with expansion of therapeutic spas. German Hospital in Istanbul operates the country's first ISO certified IVF center, while Memorial Hospital was the first private hospital to receive American JCI accreditation. According to Visit and Care, a medical tourism agency in Istanbul, average medical costs are 50%-75% lower than those in the United States.

Ukraine

Ukraine features modern dental clinics with high-quality equipment, materials and effective anesthetics. They provide patients with dentistry services at lower cost in comparison with Western and Russian clinics. Other popular medical tourism offerings in Ukraine include spas, ophthalmology (eye surgery), plastic surgery, and mud baths. As yet, Ukraine medical clinics have yet to seek international healthcare accreditation.

North America

Canada

Canada has entered the medical tourism field. In comparison to US health costs, medical tourism patients can save 30 to 60 percent on health costs in Canada. Canada's quality of healthcare is cited by the World Health Organization as equal to if not better than that of the US in most categories.

Costa Rica

Costa Rica has been actively involved with dental tourism, and US insurers have begun contracting with dentists there. Costa Rica has also recently entered the broader medical tourism market. In comparison to US health costs, medical tourism patients can save up to 80 percent on health costs in Costa Rica. In addition to dental and cosmetic procedures, orthopedic and weight-loss surgeries are rapidly becoming increasingly popular. In Costa Rica, a knee replacement surgery may cost as low as $10,500 USD compared to nearly $50,000 USD in the United States.

Recently, Clinica Biblica became the country's first JCI-accredited hospital, and is also a member of Companion Global Healthcare's network (Blue Cross Blue Shield of South Carolina) of overseas hospitals. The close proximity to the United States and Canada and a significant English speaking presence make Costa Rica a growing destination for medical travel.

Cuba

Cuba has been a popular medical tourism destination for more than 40 years. Thousands of patients travel to Cuba, particularly from Latin America and Europe, attracted by the "fine reputation of Cuban doctors, the low prices and nearby beaches on which to recuperate." In 2006, Cuba attracted nearly 20,000 health tourists.

Medical treatments included joint replacement, cancer treatment, eye surgery, cosmetic surgery and addictions rehabilitation. Costs are about 60 to 80 percent less than US costs. For example, Choice Medical Services, a health tourism provider, provides a hip replacement in Cuba for US$5,845/ C$6120/□4227.

Cuba has hospitals for Cuban residents and others that focus on serving foreigners and diplomats. In the 2007 American documentary film, "Sicko," which criticizes the US healthcare system, producer Michael Moore leads a group of uninsured American patients to Cuba to obtain more affordable medical treatment. "Sicko" has greatly increased foreigners' interest in Cuban healthcare. A recent Miami Herald story focused on the high quality of health care that Canadian and American medical tourism patients receive in Cuba.

The Cuban government has developed Cuban medical tourism to generate income for the country. Residents of Canada, the UK and most other countries can travel to Cuba without any difficulty; a tourist visa is generally required. For Americans, however, because of the US trade policy towards Cuba, travelers must either obtain US government approval, or, more frequently, travel to Cuba from Canada, Mexico, the Bahamas, Jamaica or the Dominican Republic. Cuban immigration authorities do not stamp the passports of US visitors so that Americans can keep their travels a private matter.

However, few Cuban hospitals as yet have international healthcare accreditation. None have achieved JCI Accreditation.

Dominican Republic

One of the medical tourism destinations nearest to the US mainland is the Dominican Republic. The country has become a popular destination for plastic surgeries, hip-replacements, knee replacements, bariatric surgeries, eye surgeries and all other types of surgeries and medical treatments. The costs are generally 50 to 75 percent less than cost of similar procedures in the US.

Mexico

Americans, particularly those living near the Mexican border, now routinely cross to Mexico for medical care. Popular specialties include dentristry and plastic surgery. Mexican dentists often charge one-fifth to one-fourth of US prices, while other procedures typically cost a third what they would in the US.

This trend has alarmed American healthcare providers who, fearing a loss of business, warn patients away from Mexico. "The phenomenon has unsettled US-based dentists who tell horror stories of rampant infections, undetected cases of oral cancer and shoddy work south of the border -- claims hotly disputed by Mexican dentists." "In Texas, legislators explored the possibility of allowing health maintenance organizations to operate on both sides of the border. However, physicians in south Texas lobbied against the changes, arguing that local doctors could not compete with the lower costs in Mexico". US doctors point out that the Mexican legal system makes it almost impossible to sue Mexican doctors for malpractice.

However, many who travel to Mexico for care report that they are satisfied. According to a report commissioned by Families U.S.A., a Washington advocacy group for health-care issues, "About 90 percent feel the care they had received in Mexico had been good or excellent. About 80 percent rated the care they had received in the United States as good or excellent". Indeed "some U.S. dentists ... have conceded to the competition and begun a 'reverse migration' opening offices in Mexico to take advantage of lower costs". More American insurers are providing coverage for travelers, as the out-of-pocket costs to them are much lower. "With healthcare costs in the United States continuing to rise, many employers in Southern California are turning to insurance plans that send their workers to Mexico for routine care, plans that are growing by nearly 3,000 people a year".

In addition to dental and plastic surgery, Mexican hospitals are popular for bariatric surgery for weight loss, considered an elective procedure that is not covered by some US insurers. A popular bariatric procedure, lap band surgery, which was approved by the FDA in the US in 2001, has been performed for longer by Mexican surgeons.

Panama

In Panama, health and medical tourism is growing rapidly. Factors drawing medical tourists include Panama's tourist appeal, position as a hub for international travel, and use of the dollar as the official currency. More important, Panama's medical professionals are trained around the world, use the latest technologies and medications, and have earned a high reputation.

Many of Panama's doctors are bilingual, board certified, and accustomed to working with the same medical equipment and technology used in the United States and Europe. On most procedures, Panama offers savings of more than 50% compared to the US and Europe. For example, Dental implants cost an average of $2,500 per implant in the US or Canada.

In Panama, the same procedure with board and lodging, personal tour guide, and transportation is available at a much lower cost. Popular procedures include dental implants, plastic surgery, assisted reproduction, cardiology, cosmetic dentistry, pulmonology and orthopedics. Panama's hospitals have affiliations to international organizations such as: Baptist Health International of Miami, Cleveland Clinic, Tulane Health Science Center, Johns Hopkins International, Miami Children's Hospital, University of Nebraska Medical Center, The Kendall Medical Center in Florida, and Harvard Medical Faculty and Physicians at Beth Israel Deaconess Medical Center in US.

South America

Brazil

Brazil, led by Ivo Pitanguy, has long been known as a destination for cosmetic surgery. For non-cosmetic procedures, Brazil is only now entering the global market. However, Albert Einstein Jewish Hospital in São Paulo was the first JCI-accredited facility outside of the US. The decision to obtain accreditation dates back to mid 1990s, with the goal to improve quality. In order to compete locally, other Brazilian facilities obtained accreditation, notably Hospital Samaritano and Hospital do Coração.

One advantage of Brazil for those from the US and Canada is ease of travel and relatively close proximity to North America. Brazil requires visas for Americans based on a reciprocal arrangement since Brazilians are required to obtain a visa to visit the US.

Colombia

Colombia has been treating foreign patients for years, especially for cosmetic and eye surgery. Colombia also provides advanced cardiovascular and transplant surgery. What often compels persons to seek transplant surgery offshore is not only cost considerations, but waiting lists (such as in the US) or the lack of an organized organ inventory and donor system in the home country. Colombia has such an organ donor and banking system which makes organs available to foreigners with certain legal restrictions. Orthopedic surgeries, such as knee and hip replacements, are done in Colombia with US-made, (FDA-approved) prosthetics at a fraction of the cost.

Colombia has many surgeons that have either trained and/or practiced in other countries such as the US and Europe. Salaries for doctors, nurses, and supporting personnel in Colombia are about 20% of US salaries for similar occupations even though they are required to have the same level of education and job skills. Real estate costs related to medical care facilities are also a fraction of what they are in the US. Like Brazil, ease of travel and relative proximity from the US and Canada is an advantage. Colombia offers cheaper airfares from the US and Canada (and some European countries) than other more-distant destinations, and does not have the visa restrictions of other countries currently in the medical tourism market. However, as of early 2008, no Colombian hospital has obtained JCI accreditation.

Uruguay

Uruguay recently entered the medical tourism market. The country offers internationally recognised medical professionals in one of the safest countries in Latin America, with a well-equipped infrastructure for tourists. A private medical tourism initiative, Uruhealth, has been created with support from the Ministries of Tourism and Public Health. The initiative involves the infrastructure, human resources and experience of two healthcare companies: MP Personalized Medicine (Montevideo) and SEMM-Mautone Hospital (Punta del Este).

2

Tourism for Dental Health

Dental tourism is a subset of the sector known as medical tourism. It involves individuals seeking dental care outside of their local healthcare systems.

REASONS FOR TRAVEL

While dental tourists may travel for a variety of reasons, their choices are usually driven by price considerations. Wide variations in the economics of countries with shared borders have been the historical mainstay of the sector. Examples include travel from Austria to Slovakia and Slovenia, the US to Mexico, and the Republic of Ireland to Northern Ireland. While medical tourism is often generalized to travel from high-income countries to low-cost developing economies, other factors can influence a decision to travel, including differences between the funding of public healthcare or general access to healthcare.

Mobility of Labour

For countries within the European Union, dental qualifications are required to reach a minimum approved by each country's government. Thus a dentist qualified in one country can apply to any other EU country to practice in that country, allowing for greater mobility of labour for dentists (Directives typically apply not only to the EU but to the wider designation of the European Economic Area - EEA).

The Association for Dental Education in Europe (ADEE) has standardization efforts to harmonize European standards. Proposals from the ADEE's Quality Assurance and

Benchmarking taskforce cover the introduction of accreditation procedures for EU dentistry universities as well as programmes to facilitate dental students completing part of their education in foreign dentistry schools. Standardization of qualification in a region reciprocally removes one of the perceptual barriers for the development of patient mobility within that region.

Pricing and Quality

The UK and The Republic of Ireland are two of the largest sources of dental tourists. Both have had their dental professions examined by competition authorities to determine whether consumers were receiving value for money from their dentists. Both countries' professions were criticised for a lack of pricing transparency. A response to this is that dentistry is unsuitable for transparent pricing: each treatment will vary, an accurate quote is impossible until an examination has occurred.

Procedure	United States	Mexico	Hungary
Implants, with crown	$1,000 to $5,000	$2,200	$950
Veneers	At least $1,000	$500	$360
Root canal	$360 to $1300	$450 to $500	$350
Crowns	$750 to $1,000	$500	$285
Bonding	$150 to $300	$95	$70

Thus price lists are no guarantee of final costs. Though they may encourage a level of competition between dentists, this will only happen in a competitive environment where supply and demand are closely matched. The 2007 Competition Authority report in the Irish Republic criticised the profession on its approach to increasing numbers of dentists and the training of dental specialties - orthodontics was a particular area for concern with training being irregular and limited in number of places. Supply is further limited as new dental specialties develop and dentists react to consumer demand for new dental products, further diluting the pool of dentists available for any given procedure.

MEDICAL TOURISM–HEALTH CARE IN THE GLOBAL ECONOMY

Although physician executives are certainly aware that some patients bypass their hospital, clinic or ambulatory surgery center on the way to the airport to have care in other cities, they may be somewhat surprised to learn that an increasing number of patients are traveling to a wide variety of destinations around the world for medical, surgical and dental care. Driven by a number of forces outside typical medical referral systems, these "medical tourists" seek modern health care at affordable prices in countries at variable levels of development. Medical tourism is different from the traditional form of international medical care where patients typically journey from less developed nations to major medical centers in highly developed countries for advanced medical treatment.

Popularity Growing

There is no definitive information about how many patients receive health care in the medical tourism model. A major difficulty in determining the magnitude of medical tourism is the fact that the reported numbers may include expatriates from other nations, business travelers and tourists who require medical care while they are in these destinations for other purposes. Also, ayurveda and wellness services such as yoga and massage at medi-spa resorts may be included in the tally of foreigners receiving health care. Finally, the accuracy of reported information cannot be validated. Despite these limitations, it is clear that a substantial number of patients participate in medical tourism.

In 2003, approximately 350,000 patients from industrialized nations traveled to a variety of less developed countries for health care. It is projected that 750,000 Americans will go offshore for medical care in 2007, with this number increasing to six million in 2010. In 2004, 1.18 million patients from all over the world traveled to India for health care, and Thailand cared for approximately 1.1 million medical tourists from a large number of countries in Asia, Europe and North America.

The Confederation of Indian Industry, in consultation with McKinsey and Company, reports that medical tourism in India produces annual revenue of $300 million, with projected growth to $2 billion by 2012. Articles and broadcasts on medical tourism are appearing in the press and on the airways with increasing frequency, and several guide books have been recently published. A Google Internet search on May 6, 2007 using the term "medical tourism" returned 777,000 results (Table 1).

Medical Tourism is Different

Medical tourism is market driven--it is shaped by the complex interactions of myriad medical, economic, social and political forces. Low cost is the primary reason that patients from industrialized nations seek medical care in less developed countries.

Patients in the medical tourism model would likely prefer to have major surgery in their hometown hospital or local referral center. However, these patients feel pressed to balance their health needs against other considerations; they are willing to accept uncertainties about quality in order to obtain care at prices they can more comfortably afford.

Patients from the United States typically fit one of two profiles:

1. Working class adults who require elective surgery but have no health insurance or inadequate insurance benefits
2. Patients who desire procedures not covered by insurance such as cosmetic surgery, dental reconstruction, gender reassignment operations, or fertility treatment

The key point is that resources are insufficient for them to comfortably purchase care in their local market, but adequate for them to buy care in low-cost foreign facilities.

For patients from Britain, Canada and other countries where a governmental health care system regulates access to health care, the reason to leave the local market is the desire to have timely treatment, circumventing delays associated with long waiting lists.

Because national health programs do not fund cosmetic surgery and similar type services, patients seeking these services are driven to pursue medical tourism by the same economic forces as those from the United States.

Patients also travel to medical tourism destinations for procedures that are not available in their own countries. For example, stem cell therapy for heart failure, unobtainable by many patients in industrialized countries, is available in the medical tourism marketplace.

A faraway country provides privacy and confidentiality for patients undergoing plastic surgery, sex change procedures and drug rehabilitation. Furthermore, their medical records cannot be viewed by the myriad parties who can access these documents in the United States.

There is currently virtual absence of involvement of referring physicians in medical tourism. Doctors in industrialized nations, unfamiliar with the practitioners and practices in less developed countries, are reluctant to encourage their patients to pursue care by unknown providers in distant lands.

Further, the physician may deeply believe that it is unreasonable to choose a provider for potentially risky medical therapy based on anything other than medical considerations. Finally, physicians in highly litigious nations may be particularly reluctant to endorse offshore treatment because of concern about vicarious liability.

However, there are many agencies that provide services to patients who want offshore medical and surgical care. These agencies help patients select a country, facility and provider. They determine prices and collect payment, assemble and transmit medical records, and arrange travel and accommodations. Additionally, they may arrange for postoperative follow-up in the patient's own community after they return.

Although some travel professionals promote the "tourism" aspect of offshore care, as the seriousness of the medical situation increases, the recreational aspects of travel have diminishing importance. Medical tourism agencies can be easily found on the Internet or in any medical tourism guide.

The availability of resources is the issue that most differentiates the traditional international medical patient from the patient in the medical tourism model. In the medical tourism model, the absence of some resource influences or drives the decision about travel for medical services, whereas the traditional international medical patient has ready access to health care facilities throughout the world as a consequence of available financial resources.

In the medical tourism model, poor nations export health care expertise and services to patients from industrialized countries. The direction of international trade is opposite that of the traditional model. Consequently, nations that once primarily exported medical services to less developed countries are now purchasing health care from these same countries.

The principal reason why medical tourism destinations are able to offer services so inexpensively relates to the level of their national economic development.

Accordingly, the lower cost of health care is appropriate for the economic environment in which the care is provided. Another reason for low costs overseas relates to the medicolegal environment--the professional liability insurance premium for a surgeon in India is 4 percent of what it is in New York.

Medical Tourism Destinations

Many countries are working to successfully compete in the medical tourism marketplace by offering a wide variety of medical, surgical and dental services in comfortable modern facilities.

Medical tourists travel to the four corners of the world for executive health evaluations, ophthalmologic care, cosmetic dentistry and surgery, bariatric procedures, joint resurfacing or replacement, cardiac surgery, organ and stem cell transplantation, gender reassignment surgery and in-vitro fertilization. Several countries in Central and South America have developed strong reputations for cosmetic and plastic surgery, bariatric procedures, and dental care.

Destinations in Asia are particularly popular for orthopedics and cardiac surgery. India, Singapore and Thailand are well-established medical tourism destinations, attracting large numbers of foreign patients and generating substantial revenue from the services provided. These countries have large, modern medical facilities that are staffed by well-trained physicians who perform complex procedures such as minimally invasive/ off-pump heart surgery, correction of congenital cardiac abnormalities in children, thoracic organ transplantation, and implantation of mechanical cardiac assist devices. An article in the Washington Post reports on a cardiac hospital in India that has outstanding outcomes with coronary artery bypass surgery. Thailand's international hospitals have a reputation for having modern high-tech equipment, excellent quality medical care and superior hospitality services.

India has the important advantage of lower cost than most other destinations, at approximately 10 percent of the costs in the United States. South Africa has been very successful selling medical services combined with tourism activities such as safaris.

It is important to recognize that modern well-equipped hospitals in some areas of the world concurrently serve the role of regional referral centers for patients from poor neighboring countries, while at the same time functioning as low cost medical tourism destinations for patients from highly developed countries. Several highly developed nations including Canada, Germany, Italy and Israel attract foreign patients from nations at all stages of economic development under the banner of medical tourism. Medical care is delivered with a strong service focus, including visits to tourist attractions. The medical services, costs and direction of travel associated with care in these highly developed nations are more typical of the traditional international medical services model.

SAFETY AND QUALITY OF CARE

The critical challenge for potential medical tourists is to select the best possible destination for the specific services needed. Certainly, well-trained physicians and modern, well-equipped hospitals provide high-quality care in a number of medical tourism destinations.

However, patients considering offshore medical care face a daunting task in differentiating the desirable offshore destinations from those with inadequate practitioners working in unsafe facilities. Some medical tourism agents with backgrounds in health care, and a particular focus on quality and outcomes, may be a helpful resource for patients.

Accreditation by Joint Commission International and/or the International Organization of Standardization (ISO) may provide a useful and reassuring benchmark for patients in selecting offshore medical facilities. The Joint Commission began evaluating foreign hospitals in 1999 and has accredited more than 120 hospitals in 23 countries.

There are particular concerns about the possible adverse consequences of vacation activities and travel in the postoperative period, as well as uncertainties about follow-up care. The responsibility for management and costs of complications occurring after a patient is home is an important issue that remains unresolved.

The consequences of an adverse outcome, such as a severe stroke or death, in a foreign country thousands of miles from home would be particularly difficult for the family of a patient with limited funds.

Finally, if a patient wanted to initiate litigation for an adverse outcome, the claim would have to be adjudicated in a foreign court.

RESPONSE TO MEDICAL TOURISM

The American Society of Plastic Surgeons, the first medical organization to address medical tourism, posted a briefing paper on its Web site in 2005 providing information to patients considering cosmetic surgery in foreign countries.

In 2006, other medical organizations began to pay attention to medical tourism, responding with notices on their Web sites and presentations at meetings to provide information and opinions to the public and to their membership. In June 2006, The United States Senate Special Committee on Aging held hearings on the issue of medical tourism subsequent to which the Chairman, Senator Gordon Smith, called for a task force of experts to explore the impact and safety of lower cost health care abroad.

American manufacturers and insurance companies are studying and pursuing offshore health care options in an effort to reduce health care costs. Mercer Health & Benefits, a prominent employee benefits consulting firm, has been retained by three Fortune 500 corporations to determine the feasibility of directing elective major surgery to foreign medical destinations.

Currently, Blue Shield of California and Health Net sell discounted health insurance policies that encourage patients to get most of their care in Mexico, and United Group Programs, a third-party administrator, is promoting elective surgical care in Thailand.

In West Virginia, legislation was introduced that would provide financial rebates to state employees who seek health care at medical tourism destinations. Although the original bill did not make it out of committee in 2006, the issue has been reintroduced in the 2007 legislative session (HB 2841).

Challenges and Opportunities

It is inevitable that an increasing number of health insurance plans will extend their provider networks to include selected health care institutions around the world and will provide incentives to encourage beneficiaries to use offshore facilities for expensive elective surgical procedures.

The loss of even a small number of profitable insured surgical patients could endanger the viability of some programs and institutions that provide such services. This may be particularly problematic for smaller programs and for those with a preexisting unfavorable case mix.

In an article in the New England Journal of Medicine, Millstein and Smith point out that the flight of American patients to foreign destinations for lifesaving operations is symbolically important and must be addressed by physician leaders. These authors argue that Americans going to foreign destinations for surgical care is a symptom of, and not a solution to, an affordability problem.

Their analysis suggests that offshore surgery could decrease total U.S. household spending for health care by only 1 percent to 2 percent. Mattoo (a World Bank economist) and Rathindran report that a number of health care services are readily tradable and that potential gains from trade could benefit all parties, with US health care savings of $1.4 billion to $2 billion.

Medical institutions in less developed countries benefit by serving foreign patients. The skills and financial resources derived by providing health care in the global marketplace allow these facilities to better care for the local residents who otherwise would have limited access to modern medical facilities and services.

Medical tourism enables countries that have long waiting lists for certain procedures to clear their backlog by sending patients to foreign countries for expedient care, at low cost, without expanding local capacity. Finally, there are opportunities for innovative physician executives and other health care leaders to explore ways to better fund the care of poor patients by directing certain services to lower cost hospitals in foreign destinations.

What's called medical tourism ? patients going to a different country for either urgent or elective medical procedures ? is fast becoming a worldwide, multibillion-dollar industry. The reasons patients travel for treatment vary. Many medical tourists from the United States are seeking treatment at a quarter or sometimes even a 10th of the cost at home. From Canada, it is often people who are frustrated by long waiting times. From Great Britain, the patient can't wait for treatment by the National Health Service but also can't afford to see a physician in private practice. For others, becoming a medical tourist is a chance to combine a tropical vacation with elective or plastic surgery.

And more patients are coming from poorer countries such as Bangladesh where treatment may not be available. Medical tourism is actually thousands of years old. In ancient Greece, pilgrims and patients came from all over the Mediterranean to the sanctuary of the healing god, Asklepios, at Epidaurus. In Roman Britain, patients took the waters at a shrine at Bath, a practice that continued for 2,000 years. From the 18th century wealthy Europeans travelled to spas from Germany to the Nile. In the 21st century, relatively low-cost jet travel has taken the industry beyond the wealthy and desperate.

Countries that actively promote medical tourism include Cuba, Costa Rica, Hungary, India, Israel, Jordan, Lithuania, Malaysia and Thailand. Belgium, Poland and Singapore are now entering the field. South Africa specializes in medical safaris-visit the country for a safari, with a stopover for plastic surgery, a nose job and a chance to see lions and elephants. India is considered the leading country promoting medical tourism-and now it is moving into a new area of "medical outsourcing," where subcontractors provide services to the overburdened medical care systems in western countries.

India's National Health Policy declares that treatment of foreign patients is legally an "export" and deemed "eligible for all fiscal incentives extended to export earnings." Government and private sector studies in India estimate that medical tourism could bring between $1 billion and $2 billion US into the country by 2012. The reports estimate that medical tourism to India is growing by 30 per cent a year. India's top-rated education system is not only churning out computer programmers and engineers, but an estimated 20,000 to 30,000 doctors and nurses each year.

The largest of the estimated half-dozen medical corporations in India serving medical tourists is Apollo Hospital Enterprises, which treated an estimated 60,000 patients between 2001 and spring 2004. It is Apollo that is aggressively moving into medical outsourcing. Apollo already provides overnight computer services for U.S. insurance companies and hospitals as well as working with big pharmaceutical corporations with drug trials. Dr. Prathap C. Reddy, the chairman of the company, began negotiations in the spring of 2004 with Britain's National Health Service to work as a subcontractor, to do operations and medical tests for patients at a fraction of the cost in Britain for either government or private care.

Apollo's business began to grow in the 1990s, with the deregulation of the Indian economy, which drastically cut the bureaucratic barriers to expansion and made it easier to import the most modern medical equipment. The first patients were Indian expatriates who returned home for treatment; major investment houses followed with money and then patients from Europe, the Middle East and Canada began to arrive. Apollo now has 37 hospitals, with about 7,000 beds. The company is in partnership in hospitals in Kuwait, Sri Lanka and Nigeria. Western patients usually get a package deal that includes flights, transfers, hotels, treatment and often a post-operative vacation.

Apollo has also reacted to criticism by Indian politicians by expanding its services to India's millions of poor. It has set aside free beds for those who can't afford care, has set up a trust fund and is pioneering remote, satellite-linked telemedicine across India.

In a country as diverse and complex as India, it is not surprising to find that people here reflect the rich glories of the past, the culture, traditions and values relative to geographic locations and the numerous distinctive manners, habits and food that will always remain truly Indian.

Beaches in India

Thousands of sun-deprived tourists visit India because it incredibly has the most diverse varieties of beaches anywhere in the world. Placid backwaters and lagoons, bays and rough lava-rocked seas, marine estuaries with fish, crashing surf, powdery golden sand or palm fringed shores - Incredible India has them all. The West Coast with the Arabian Sea and the East Coast with the Bay of Bengal offer many a verdant vistas to the traveller. The coasts of India have their own seafood cuisine, relaxing spas, diving and water sports and great places to stay for a balmy holiday.

Hill Stations and Retreats

India offers several Hill Stations with excellent tourist attractions and facilities.

Royal Retreats

Having had a glorious past ranging from old civilizations to the more recent kingdoms, India offers royal retreats which are nowhere to be seen elsewhere. Staying at beautiful palaces with lush green fields, huge borders etc., make some of these retreats a memory of a lifetime.

Medical Packages

The health care sector in India has witnessed an enormous growth in infrastructure in the private and voluntary sector. The private sector which was very modest in the early stages, has now become a flourishing industry equipped with the most modern state-of-the-art technology at its disposal. It is estimated that 75-80% of health care services and investments in India are now provided by the private sector. An added plus had been that India has one of the largest pharmaceutical industries in the world. It is self sufficient in drug production and exports drugs to more than 180 countries.

- Bone Marrow Transplant
- Brain Surgery
- Cancer Procedures (Oncology)
- Cardiac Care
- Cosmetic Surgery
- Dialysis and Kidney Transplant
- Drug Rehabilitation
- Gynaecology & Obstetrics
- Health Checkups
- Internal/Digestive Procedures
- Joint Replacement Surgery
- Nuclear Medicine
- Neurosurgery & Trauma Surgery

- Preventive Health Care
- Refractive Surgery
- Osteoporosis
- Spine Related
- Urology
- Vascular Surgery

Hi-Tech Healing Opportunities in India

The health care sector in India has witnessed an enormous growth in infrastructure in the private and voluntary sector. The private sector, which was very modest in the early stages, has now become a flourishing industry equipped with the most modern state-of-the-art technology at its disposal. It is estimated that 75-80 per cent of health care services and investment in India are now provided sector.An added plus has been that India has one of the largest pharmaceutical industries in the world. It is self sufficient in drug production and exports drugs to more than 180 countries.

The privatization of the medicare sector has brought with it five-star facilities and world-class treatments. The country can now boast of a number of corporate hospitals. India is a source market for professionals in the medical field for most of the renowned hospitals around the world. Hi-tech medical facilities have become a necessity following consumer demand among the world's fastest growing middle class. India offers at its own doorstep, a range of world quality hospitals and treatments at a fraction of world costs with comparable success rates and service levels directly in proportion to the high value system and natural caring that comes with its millennia heritage. Indian hospitals are becoming known internationally for standards of health care delivery, comparable to the best in the world. India has the technology and the skilled super specialists coupled with sound infrastructure and professional management, nurses and paramedical staff to take on international competition.

Health Tourism is a concept where a patient travels to another country for medical treatment in order to save costs, or get treatment faster or even to avail of better medical facilities. Most patients from countries like USA and UK travel to developing countries such as India for treatment because India offers some of te cheapest pricing options of treatment, offers a good holiday, there are no waiting lists or queues to stand in, the doctors are comparable to anyone in the world and finally, language does not pose a problem as most people speak English.

Why would Someone Travel to India and not to Thailand?

Although the cost difference between treatment in India and Thailand is not much, India offers what you call a language advantage - a patient would surely prefer a country where English is widely spoken. Also, it is believed that the facilities in India are more suited for International patients. India is also working hard to increase it's infrastructure to better suit the needs of patients coming to India for treatments such as heart surgey, knee replacement, other orthopaedic treatments, cosmetic surgery, eye care, dental treatment or any other treatment for that matter. This is one of the primary fields which India intends to explore during the coming years.

How can you Trust Indian Doctors?

Well, many highly qualified doctors have had some form of training from abroad , specially USA and UK. Indian surgeons and doctors are known for their skill and research throughout the world. India has over 150000 medical tourists each year and this figure is rising at a high pace. Some recent programs recently on BBC and CNBC have reinstated the fact that medical tourism is a good idea if - you want to save costs, you need the treatment to be done at your time and convenience, you need a high quality budget incorporated.

More and more people have started travelling to India for Medical Treatment and during the past year alone, over 150000 people travelled to India for their medical requirements. Medical Tourism is finally coming of age. India boasts of several good private owned hospitals with facilities second to none. They have some of the best doctors, with most top end being educated in USA and UK. When it comes to becoming a doctor, India also has some of the stringest criteria. Language is another plus factor - English, which is widely spoken throughout the country and in all good hospitals. Furthermore, the costs are much lower than most countries and most importantly, there are no waiting lists. With all the media hype about medical tourism, most hospitals have geared themselves up for medical tourists from abroad.

Medical Tourism companies in India such as Health Line - http://www.indiamedicaltourism.net have introduced several packages for patients travelling to India which include holidays and hotel stays during their travel apart from other basic requirements such as airport pickup, meetings with doctors post and pre-surgery etc. Such packages make it convenient for the patient to have peace of mind during travel without the tension of what to do next. For all those still hesitant to travel abroad for treatment, try getting a package deal with a company such as Health Line and you will get an idea of how much you can save.

No coss are incurred for getting a quote or medical advise over email. Doctors are very willing to help patients abroad feel comfortable and will be more than happy to respond to your queries through such medical tourism companies. With the introduction of the medical visa, it will now be easier than ever to travel to India. If your treatment requires an extension, the medical visa can be extended without any problem. Ending on one final note, do not forget to include your medical reports before travelling to India. Heart Treatment in India costs much lower than traditional hospitals in developed countries and in most cases, lower than other developing countries.

They use some of the best technology and knowhow and the procedures include cardiothoracic, neurology, gastrointestinal, orthopaedic, renal, obstetric, ENT, opthalmology, dental, plastic, cosmetic and tumour surgeries. The cost difference can be as high as 1:3, which effectively means you get a 5 star treatment at one-third the costs using top class doctors. Leave alone the cost, there is no queue, no waiting lists and you will get preferential treatment. Conditions operated on include:

Heart Care

—Valvular diseases

—Arrhythmias

—Coronary artery disease

—Hypercholesterolemia

—Family history of coronary disease

—Hypercholesterolemia

—Heart disease symptoms

Table : Results of Internet Search for Terms Related to Medical Tourism.

Search term	Number of Internet sites identified
"medical tourism"	777,000
"medical tourism" + surgery	239,000
"medical tourism" + heart	169,000
"medical tourism" + heart + surgery	111,000
"medical tourism" + cardiac + surgery	121,000
"medical tourism" + transplantation	81,900
"medical tourism" + cancer	152,000
"medical tourism" + obesity	85,400
"medical tourism" + bariatric	24,600
"medical tourism" + joint	86,700
"medical tourism" + hip	79,200
"medical tourism" + prostate	62,400
"medical tourism" + cosmetic	123,000
"medical tourism" + plastic + surgery	136,000
"medical tourism" + dentistry	189,000
"medical tourism" + surgery + sex	51,300
"medical tourism" + savings	67,600

Some of the procedures available are:

—directional coronary atherectomy

—rotablation

—coronary artery stenting

—intravascular ultrasound

—balloon valvuloplasty

—non-surgical closure of holes in the heart such as ASD, VSD and PDA.

It is commonly known that most top Indian doctors have top class education including training/education from Americal institutions. Add to that the world class technology and 5 star facilities and what you have is a more convenient option with an almost free holiday (keeping in mind you have significant cost savings).

(a) GoogleTM, May 6, 2007.

Reasons patients seek care at medical tourism destinations.

1. Low cost

* No insurance/inadequate insurance

—Particularly patients from United States

* Plastic and cosmetic surgery

* Cosmetic dentistry/extensive dental reconstruction

* Bariatric surgery and subsequent body contouring

* Gender reassignment procedures

* Treatment of infertility

2. Avoid waiting lists

* Countries with National Health Service

—Particularly patients from Britain and Canada

3. Procedure not available in home country

* Newly developed procedures not approved by regulatory agencies

—Stem cell therapy

—Joint resurfacing

—Artificial disc replacement (multi-level)

* Procedures unavailable or restricted by society and/or legal system

—Organ transplantation

—In-vitro fertilization with donor eggs

4. Tourism and vacations

* Luxurious accommodations and excellent service

* Exotic vacation destinations

5. Privacy and confidentiality

• ***Table : Medical tourism destinations.***[a]

Asia	The Americas	Europe	Africa
China	Argentina	Belgium	South Africa
India	Bolivia	Germany	
Israel	Brazil	Hungary	Australia
Jordan	Colombia	Lithuania	
Singapore	Costa Rica	Poland	
Malaysia	Cuba		
Philippines	Jamaica		
United Arab Emirates	Mexico		
	United States (b)		

(a) Most frequently identified countries in literature and Internet search.

(b) Leigh S. Reproductive 'tourism'. USA Today May 2, 2005.

3

Philippines Medical Tourism

Medical tourism in the Philippines is the practice of travelling to Cebu, Philippines to have a medical, dental, or surgical procedure performed, while at the same time touring, vacationing, and enjoying the country. Most often the medical procedure is an elective one that is not immediately required under time limits. The most common of these elective, non-time sensitive procedures in Cebu are dermatology (skin related), cosmetic or aesthetic surgery, routine dental services, aesthetic dental procedures, weight loss surgery, and opthalmology (eyesight related). There are 2 primary reasons that you should consider medical tourism in the Philippines.

The high cost of healthcare in industrialized countries is often 10 or more times the cost of the same procedure in Cebu. And the recent advances and improvements in technology has increased the standard of care available. Also, there is a time factor that you neeed to consider if you live in a country with socialized healthcare such as Canada or some of the EU countries. Some medical procedures in these countries may require a wait of a year or more. In Cebu, you can arrive on a certain day and within 2 or 3 days have the procedure performed.

WHY HAVE COSMETIC SURGERY?

There is no doubt that most cultures are youth centered. Maintaining a youthful appearance helps you in many ways.

The most obvious advantage in maintaining a youthful appearance is your appeal to the opposite sex. Whether you are single or married, attraction of your partner or potential partners is important to maintaining that magnetic sex appeal. Looking good also helps you feel good about yourself! Studies have also shown that good looks are a factor in earning more money and receiving promotions at work.

WHY MEDICAL TOURISM IN THE PHILIPPINES?

Cebu clearly has many advantages as a medical tourist destination. English is widely spoken in Cebu and is the primary language of instruction in all of the universities. Also, Filipinos have a natural tendency as excellent caregivers. This is partly due to the fact that there are no nursing homes here to care for the elderly, consequently family members must care for their parents and grandparents. The low cost of the medical procedures, accommodations, food and transportation in Cebu make it a very attractive destination. There are also a large number of spas and massage centers to facilitate recovery and relaxation. Finally, the medical staff often consists of personnel that have been trained in the U.S., Japan, or Singapore. All in all, medical tourism in the Philippines, specifically Cebu, has several advantages to the medical tourist. So, come to the wellness island of Cebu and look good, feel good, and have a good time!

The Philippines offers visitors traveling to the country for medical treatment high standards in care and services, while also providing a paradisiacal holiday destination for pre- and post treatment relaxation. Many of the top hospitals which entice medical visitors with their range of excellent procedures at prices far below those in developed countries are located close to some of the most popular tourist spots. The medical tourism industry in the Philippines has grown at a remarkable rate in recent years, with more hospitals being established outside the country's capital, particularly in central provinces such as Luzon and Davao. Americans facing increasingly rising costs for medical treatments are some of the Philippines' most important customers, while those traveling from Europe also make up a decent percentage of medical customers here. Among the most popular treatments are cosmetic and plastic surgery, weight loss surgery and dental procedures. In addition, more serious operations such as artery bypass surgery and kidney transplant are slowly drawing more visitors. State of the art facilities, highly trained medical staff and the unique Filipino hospitality are among the most enticing reasons to make a medical trip to this Asian paradise.

It is primarily the low cost of high level service that sees Europeans and Americans disregard the medical offerings in their home countries. By coming to the Philippines for surgery, they are also faced with the opportunity not only to have procedures carried out at a saving, but also to holiday in an exotic location. Spa resorts, pristine beaches and excellent tour infrastructure mean medical tourists can take advantage of the Philippines' rapidly developing tourism industry.

Philippine Herbal Plant and the Island of Fire

When searching for a Philippine herbal plant the more adventurous can visit the Island of Fire, commonly known as Siquijor. Filipinos know Siquijor as the mystic island. Feared by many Filipinos for its sorcerers, known locally as "mambabarangs," the island has also earned a reputation for the apparently incredible powers of its local healers, or "mananambals". A 30-minute ferry ride from Dumaguete City on central Negros Island, the tiny, pristine island skirted by white beaches and surrounded by turquoise blue water has become a major draw for believers and the curious alike.

From the rich and famous to the curious, Siquijor is attracting Filipinos and foreigners -- especially around Easter -- for what is commonly referred to as the "Witches Festival" when people buy potions for everything from improving their sex life to curing terminal illnesses. The healers begin collecting the Philippine herbal plant and various plants and sea creatures that go into their potions each Friday after Ash Wednesday, 40 days before Good Friday. On Good Friday they will have gathered everything they need to make potions for the coming year, and on Saturday they start to chop and mix the ingredients.

Nothing will be collected again until Ash Wednesday the following year. The 10 medicinal plants described below are defined as a Philippine herbal plant that the Philippine Department of Health, through its "Traditional Health Program", has endorsed. All 10 herbs have been tested and have been clinically proven to have medicinal value in the relief and treatment of various aliments:

1. Akapulko (Cassia alata) - also known as "bayabas-bayabasan" and "ringworm bush" in English, this herbal medicine is used to treat ringworms and skin fungal infections.
2. Ampalaya (Momordica charantia) - known as "bitter gourd" or "bitter melon" in English, it's mostly known as a treatment of diabetes (diabetes mellitus), for the non-insulin dependent patients.
3. Bawang (Allium sativum) - popularly known as "garlic", it mainly reduces cholesterol in the blood and hence, helps control blood pressure.
4. Bayabas (Psidium guajava) - "guava" in English. It is primarily used as an antiseptic, to disinfect wounds. Also, it can be used as a mouth wash to treat tooth decay and gum infection.
5. Lagundi (Vitex negundo) - known in English as the "5-leaved chaste tree". It's main use is for the relief of coughs and asthma.
6. Niyog-niyogan (Quisqualis indica L.) - is a vine known as "Chinese honey suckle". It is effective in the elimination of intestinal worms, particularly the Ascaris and Trichina. Only the dried matured seeds are medicinal -crack and ingest the dried seeds two hours after eating (5 to 7 seeds for children & 8 to 10 seeds for adults). If one dose of the Philippine herbal plant does not eliminate the worms, wait a week before repeating the dose.
7. Sambong (Blumea balsamifera)- English name: Blumea camphora. A diuretic that helps in the excretion of urinary stones. It can also be used as an edema.

8. Tsaang Gubat (Ehretia microphylla Lam.) - Prepared like tea, this Philippine herbal plant is effective in treating intestinal motility and also used as a mouth wash since the leaves of this shrub have high fluoride content.
9. Ulasimang Bato (Peperomia pellucida) - also known as "pansit-pansitan" it is effective in fighting arthritis and gout. The leaves can be eaten fresh (about a cupful) as salad or like tea. For the decoction, boil a cup of clean chopped leaves in 2 cups of water. Boil for 15 to 20 minutes. Strain, let cool and drink a cup after meals (3 times day).
10. Yerba Buena (Clinopodium douglasii) - commonly known as Peppermint, this vine is used as an analgesic to relive body aches and pain. It can be taken internally as a decoction or externally by pounding the leaves and applied directly on the afflicted area.

Rising popularity of medical tourism reveals deterioration of U.S. healthcare system. Defenders of organized medicine are fond of saying that the United States has the best healthcare in the world, but I challenge that. I don't think we have the best healthcare in the world, I think we have the most expensive healthcare in the world. In fact, in terms of results for dollars spent, I think the United States ranks very near the bottom of the list of all industrialized nations. We get less actual health than anyone else for each dollar that we spend.

This realization is now hitting the general public as well, and they are increasingly leaving this country to find offshore locations and assess quality medical care and surgical procedures elsewhere. This phenomenon is called "medical tourism."

In medical tourism, patients who might normally undergo some sort of medical procedure in the United States, usually a costly surgical procedure, instead fly to the Philippines, Thailand or other countries to have the procedures done there.

As a result, they save an enormous amount of money. Offshore medical procedures can be performed for as little as one-tenth the cost of what would normally be charged here in the United States. And yet the facilities offshore are state of the art. These are modern hospitals that often are newer and have much better technology and equipment than hospitals in the United States. They are typically staffed by Western doctors and surgeons trained in Western medicine, and they provide equal or greater quality surgical care than U.S. hospitals. These surgical procedures are performed with the same technology and expertise, yet cost a fraction of the price.

For example, a knee replacement surgery in a high-tech hospital in the Philippines performed by Western trained surgeons might only cost you $6,000. Here in the United States you're probably looking at $50,000. Heart bypass surgery in Asia costs around $10,000. In the US, it's $60,000 to $80,000. Gastric bypass surgery in the U.S. can cost $10,000 to $20,000. Overseas it can be done for well under $5,000.

So where do the cost savings come from? How come these hospitals offshore can offer these services at much lower prices? The answer lies in the economics of healthcare in the United States and the amount of fraud and waste that is present in the U.S. healthcare system. I've spoken to many MDs over the years, and some insist that as much as 80% of all healthcare dollars that go through their office cover nothing but paperwork.

Many workers in the health care industry are basically getting paid to shuffle paper around. The health insurance companies are paid to deny health claims and the government workers at Medicare and Medicaid offices are paid to find new ways to deny payments to doctors and hospitals for services rendered. Thus, doctors' offices and hospitals have to employ entire armies of people to sit around and reclassify procedures in ways that can get paid by insurance companies, Medicare and Medicaid. It's a massive waste of time, money and effort.

In the U.S. healthcare system, it's a paperwork nightmare. And there is a paperwork war taking place. All of this is a result of health insurance, both taxpayer-funded health insurance and private health insurance. In other words, things would be a lot simpler if people just price-shopped some of these procedures and paid out of their own pocket, rather than having to go through a monstrous bureaucratic system of paper shufflers.

As a medical tourist in another country, you eliminate these paperwork shufflers. And right there, you can save as much as 80% right off the bat. Because now, your dollars are actually going to the surgeons, anesthesiologists and other hospital workers who are attending to you during your surgical procedure. Whereas in the United States, your money is going to the insurance company and then the insurance company money is being used to pay paper shufflers.

Another reason these surgical procedures are so much more affordable in Asia or the Philippines is because of the liability issue. In the United States, doctors and hospitals must carry extremely expensive medical malpractice insurance policies. And patients seem to love to sue in the United States. In contrast, when you undergo a surgical procedure as a medical tourist in an offshore hospital, you sign paperwork that says you agree not to sue under certain conditions. Thus, you save a fortune by essentially not funding the legal fees, settlements and malpractice insurance costs normally found in a U.S.-based healthcare practice. When you combine these two savings - the paperwork shuffling reduction and the medical malpractice lawsuits - and you get an incredible deal for your dollar.

Some people might ask, "What if something goes wrong during the surgery?" Well, here you have the reputation of the hospital and the surgeon at stake. They know that they must offer you outstanding, high-quality service. Otherwise, word will spread via the internet and elsewhere, and tourists won't come visit their hospital.

Medical tourism hospitals in the Philippines and other countries actually have to meet a higher standard, because they know there's more on the line. They have to give you such a high-quality experience with such outstanding results that you go back home to the United States and tell 20 people. Because when you do that, they know they're going to get more customers, and this is great word of mouth marketing for that hospital.

They're going to do their absolute best to make sure that you have a wonderful experience. Whereas in the United States, that incentive is not in place. Many hospitals realize they won't be paid much for your procedure because of all the paperwork shuffling and the late payments by insurance companies and Medicare. So they have no incentive to have more patients come in with low-quality insurance. And besides, they've probably got patients coming in through the door every single day anyway, so there's really no incentive to give you an outstanding, positive experience. At least it's not the same incentive offered by these outsourced, offshore medical facilities that base their very existence on reputation and word of mouth.

All this doesn't mean something can't go wrong, because we are of course talking about Western medicine and surgical procedures. Things can go wrong, but they can go wrong anywhere. Something like one percent of all people undergoing gastric bypass surgery die on the operating table. That's going to happen in any country, anywhere you are. And whether or not there's medical insurance and malpractice insurance in effect at the time of your surgery doesn't affect your outcome. All it does is it gives people a chance to sue when they don't get the outcome they want.

Personally, I'm against radical Western surgical procedures to begin with, especially things like gastric bypass surgery. I think surgery should only be a last resort, and should never be used to treat chronic diseases like obesity, cancer, diabetes or heart disease. I think surgery is really only appropriate in very rare cases of those diseases, or when treating trauma and accident patients. In those cases, surgery is well justified and greatly needed.

So I am not at all a proponent of Western-style surgical procedures, but if you are going to get them done, I think you're going to have much better results by checking out medical tourism and going to hospitals overseas, where you get the same or better care at a fraction of the price you'd be paying here in the United States. Plus you get a vacation out of it, too. So if you get your knee replaced at a hospital in Thailand, you can take a tour before or after the surgery and soak up a little bit of Southeast Asia culture. Learn something about what it's like in Thailand before you undergo your surgical procedure. That can be a healing experience all by itself.

But getting back to the popularity of medical tourism, we're seeing this come on with strong momentum right now. More and more people are taking this option. They're booking tickets, going online to learn more about these hospitals, and opting to have these surgical procedures done overseas.

This is very bad news for the U.S. healthcare industry, because for a long time, healthcare was an industry that people thought could be protected here in the United States. As jobs were lost overseas in the Information Technology, accounting and technical support industries, people thought, "Well, that's manageable, but no one will go overseas to have medical care." It turns out they were wrong. People will go overseas to get better medical care or a better value on surgical procedures, and the popularity of medical tourism is proving that.

What it could mean long term is a further deterioration of the U.S. healthcare system. If healthcare becomes so expensive in this country that it's by far cheaper to buy an international plane ticket and get some medical procedure done overseas, then more and more people are going to take that option and go overseas.

So in addition to exporting so many jobs from the IT industry, we will actually be exporting healthcare revenues to countries around the world. And these are substantial revenues; we're talking about billions of dollars at stake. In fact, many of these Asian countries are counting on this revenue as an increasingly important part of their Gross Domestic Product. Some of these countries are saying tourism is big and medical tourism is going to be big. And they're putting a lot of money into building state-of-the-art infrastructure and engaging in marketing to attract more medical tourists.

It's a very big deal to these countries. They see the opportunity and they see the U.S. healthcare system stumbling. Meanwhile, Americans are getting more diseased than ever before, so there's an instant customer base for hospitals around the world who can offer quality care at a better price. The U.S., for its part, tends to be rather protectionist about all of this. We've seen, for example, the FDA seizing the importation of perfectly legal prescription drugs because it doesn't want drugs to come into this country. It wants to protect the U.S. pharmaceutical industry and make sure that customers have to buy prescription drugs here in the United States at monopoly prices. That's a protectionist philosophy that goes against every free market economic principle we've known to be true in this world.

Similarly, the FDA wants to regulate and even outlaw most nutritional supplements and medicinal herbs. That's once again a protectionist strategy to protect the profits of the pharmaceutical industry. I wouldn't be surprised if sooner or later someone in organized medicine argues that outsourcing our offshore surgical procedures is hurting the U.S. economy, and they might try to pass a law that makes it illegal to go overseas to get surgery. There have already been many attempts to arrest people traveling to anti-cancer clinics in Mexico, or to seize their medicinal herbs as they come back across the border.

There is a Gestapo-like effort out there to try to shut down anything that tries to compete with the overpriced, ineffective U.S. healthcare system. And as medical tourism becomes more popular, I think we're going to see the American Medical Association, hospital associations and maybe even the FDA up in arms, complaining about the loss of revenue to U.S. companies. Because, let's face it: big medicine is big business. And organize medicine absolutely hates competition.

I say you can't stop the free market. When people find out about medical tourism, they're going to get information on the internet, make informed decisions, go overseas and get high-quality care at a fraction of the price they'd be paying in the United States. And they're going to come back and tell lots of people.

As a nation, you can outlaw that, but all you're going to do is criminalize citizens of our society who should never be criminalized. They're just seeking honest, affordable health care. They just want a procedure that they can afford. I mean, some families have had their insurance dropped when they're facing, for example, a heart bypass surgery. They can't shell out six figures here in the United States. Is it justified to outlaw the practice of medical tourism, and force that family to skip that surgical procedure because they don't have the money to pay for it here in the United States? Maybe that family only has $10,000. Well, that means they could probably afford that procedure somewhere else. Shouldn't they have the right to make that choice and go where they want?

These are some interesting arguments that will come up. And I think it's very dangerous for any government to start telling its citizens where they can travel and for what reasons they can travel. When you have restrictions on travel, restrictions on nutritional supplements and restrictions on people buying drugs from Canada, you begin to see a sharp deterioration of freedom in this country. You lose freedom and you become more of a police state. That's what we're seeing in this country today.

All of that stands at odds with the fact that we live in a global economy. We must be able to compete globally from this point on, and if we cannot compete globally and have a more efficient healthcare system that eliminates the fraud waste and the paperwork waste, and if we do not have a more efficient tax system such as the flat tax, we're going to pay the price in this country. In terms of healthcare, people are going to go somewhere else to get it. People are going to go somewhere else to buy their prescription drugs.

(And in terms of the flat tax, investors with billions of dollars are going to put their money in other countries because the money flows where the tax code is simplified. If you want to attract billions of dollars of investments to the United States, simplify the tax code and convert to a flat tax. We will have prosperity like we've never witnessed before, because billions of dollars around the world will come flowing into this country to create new jobs and invest in new businesses.) And if you want to have a healthcare system that works in this country, you need to make it efficient. You need to get rid of the paperwork, the fraud and the waste, and have a system that offers medical procedures at a fair, affordable price. People around the world should be coming to the United States to get their surgeries done -- if we had the best healthcare system in the world. But that is no longer the case. It was true 20 years ago, but today Americans are leaving the U.S. to have their surgeries done in Asia.

That's the story on medical tourism, and it's yet another demonstration of the deterioration of the U.S. healthcare system and the failure of organized medicine.

Medical tourism, as it is now known, is a growing industry and more and more countries are jumping on the bandwagon to offer people competitively priced elective surgery, cosmetic surgery and dentistry abroad. The reasons for choosing to travel abroad for medical treatment are different for everyone but with lengthy NHS waits and concerns about MRSA in NHS hospitals there is little wonder that a growing number of Brits are taking advantage of affordable, high quality private healthcare abroad, and combining it with a tropical, cultural or relaxing holiday on a Caribbean island, in a cultural European capital, or the south of Spain, saving thousands of pounds compared with having the treatment done privately in the UK.

Read all you can and talk to people who have been abroad for surgery to help make your decision Scan the newspapers or TV to see which countries are getting good press for their medical expertise. India's health care sector, for example, has undergone an enormous boom in recent years and has become a global health destination offering some of the best medical treatment in the world, despite the perceived shortcomings of healthcare in developing countries.

Meanwhile closer to home, European countries like Belgium, Hungary and Poland are offering excellent cosmetic dentistry and cosmetic surgery treatments for reasonable prices, and are only a short flight from the UK. Look out for exhibitions on medical tourism and meet international healthcare providers at events such as India's Medical Tourism Expo in London or Turkey's Healthex London Exhibition (February 2007).

However medical tourism does not appeal to all; decide whether being away from your home and family to have surgery/ treatment would bother you, do you often feel home-sick when holidaying abroad? If you feel it could be for you, then find out what you need to consider.

What to Consider?

Find out as much as possible about the procedure you are interested in - an informed patient is more able to make an informed decision. With cosmetic surgery and cosmetic dentistry different techniques and materials may be used for different procedures, so find out which method and materials are used by the provider. It is imperative that you compare services, treatments, costs and credentials of providers (see the Treatment Abroad web site - www.treatmentabroad.net - for cost comparisons and read some of the patient stories on the web site for an insight into other people's experiences.

Think about how long you want to go away for and how far you are prepared to travel. Will you have to go alone, or will a close friend/member of the family be able to accompany you? (Some providers often provide escorts for those traveling alone). Try to be as flexible with your schedule as you can as you may have to stay longer if there is a complication, and it is preferable that the surgeon and provider treat you there and then, rather than at home when it becomes more difficult.

However tantalising the prospect of cosmetic surgery in an exotic country like Malaysia or South Africa sounds, will you be comfortable on a long flight and would your doctor deem you fit for traveling long distance? Don't let the allure of a holiday in an exciting destination you haven't visited before become more important than the reputation of the surgery/dentistry/ medical treatment in that particular country.

Having an operation/surgery closer to home can be advantageous. if you decide to return for further treatment or if it is necessary to go back for follow ups - it will be much cheaper and easier to do this in Europe than a far flung destination.

Deciding where to Go

Each country varies in terms of savings, costs and areas of surgical specialty. Within Europe, Poland and Hungary are popular destinations for low cost dentistry, Belgium for cosmetic and elective surgery, and France attracts patients for obesity surgery, orthopedic and heart surgery. Even with the cost of flights to exotic places such as Malaysia and Venezuela, the savings are still beneficial and can often outweigh the cost of surgery alone in the UK - and you get to enjoy a holiday in a country you may not have been to before.

Find out if the intended procedure is available in your chosen country. There are different types of healthcare providers from major hospitals to smaller clinics and private practices, so decide which you would prefer, and whether you want to deal directly with the provider, or go through a company working as a medical tourism tour operator (an agent or broker), who will arrange the full trip abroad, putting you in touch with recommended health providers and organising your medical care, accommodation and travel within a lump-sum package.

If you are going directly to the provider make initial contact via their website or by telephone to enquire about the surgery you are interested in. Ask for some literature and brochures detailing more information about costs and the surgeon's professional background etc.

Find out all you can about the hospital/clinic's reputation - the more you know, the more prepared you are. Ask if initial consultations and follow ups can be done in the UK as some doctors come to the UK periodically to visit patients. If so, check whether the consultation in the UK will be with the same surgeon to perform the operation, or with a nurse or advisor. Seeing the surgeon / dentist for a consultation locally will give you a better understanding of what is involved and a good consultation will inform you of what the surgeon believes are the best procedures for you as well as outlining any possible risks and complications. If it isn't possible to meet the consultant locally you should ask to speak to them on the phone or email and ask as many questions as you like. Have your medical history to hand when you do so. Check whether after the operation you will stay in the hospital or be discharged and taken to a hotel; ask about special care or assistance after the procedure and about contingency plans in case of complications during the procedure or recovery time.

Do they recommend having a close friend or family member travel with you to provide support?

Find out when the country's high season is so that you can avoid exorbitant flight prices and enjoy more moderate weather.

Be honest with yourself about the importance of going to a country where fluent English is spoken and choose your destination accordingly as some medical staff in clinics and hospitals abroad do speak fluent English, while others hire translators.

Read up on local costs, the prices of meals, transport and hotels, how easy is it to travel around and whether it is considered safe to do so. The Foreign Office website will help with this and provides tips on traveling abroad with its Know Before You Go campaign.

Comparing the Costs

Get quotes from the healthcare provider or medical tourism agent/broker; many offer surgery packages including flights, accommodation and transfers. Look up the country's currency and exchange rate so you have an idea of how far your money will go in the country of choice. With so many budget airlines around, the medical tourism experience can be very affordable. During low season, return flights to Hungary can be purchased for as little as £40 with no frills airlines such as Sky Europe or Wizz Air and even with more far flung destinations such as India the overall cost can be extremely affordable - return flights are advertised from £455 with British Airways to Delhi and Mumbai and substantial savings are still made because surgery is so competitive....and of course your money goes a long way in India with around 80 Rupees to £1.

In most cases you will find there are good savings to be made by going abroad for treatment, and the cost will be cheaper than having the same procedure carried out privately in the UK. Take a look at the price comparisons on Treatment Abroad - www.treatmentabroad.net. As an example, the typical cost of Rhinoplasty (nose reshaping) in Croatia, Egypt or Turkey is around £1,500, compared with between £3,000 and £4,000 in the UK, while in India, Rhinoplasty will cost just £850.

Many of the providers will collect patients from the airport and chauffeur them to their hotel and collect them for hospital appointments, so find out whether this will be the case, and if not read up on your selected country's travel section to find out about its public transport systems and the various costs for this.

When speaking to the provider or medical broker always make sure you fully understand exactly what is included in the cost, as low prices may be offered and then extras could be added on afterwards. Ask what happens regarding the cost if a complication arises. Prices vary from provider to provider but they can typically include surgeon fees, hospital fees, medical team, hospital meals, laboratory tests, anaesthesia, implants (if appropriate), all consultations, all transfers (airport and hospital), medication, local mobile phone use and English speaking personal assistant.

In your negotiations with the provider/broker establish the means of payment. Will they require payment in advance, and/ or a deposit? Do they accept credit card, money transfers, or do they want cash payments? Is it possible to pay by installment? Before handing over any money ensure you see a valid contract first. Get everything clarified beforehand and factor in the cost of passport and/or travel visas, flights, airport pick-up, travel to-and-from medical provider, accommodation, food and drink including any tips, phone calls and other correspondence with family at home, medications or medical supplies such as crutches for hip/knee patients which may be needed post-op.

Checking out the Surgeon/dentist

Making sure that you have chosen the right surgeon or dentist begins with finding out about the qualifications and accreditations the dentists, doctors and surgeons should have in order to be practising in their country, and secondly checking that the professionals you will be seeing have these in place. Often surgeons and dentists working abroad train and qualify in the UK and if that is the case then practising doctors will be listed on the General Medical Council's (GMC) register. Cosmetic surgeons may be members of the British Association of Plastic, Reconstructive and Aesthetic Surgeons (BAPRAS) and cosmetic dentists may be listed on the General Dental Council's (GDC) register or may be members of the British Academy of Cosmetic Dentistry (BACD).

Many countries have similar associations which regulate the qualification and accreditation of surgeons and dentists. For example, the Belgian Society for Plastic Surgery is equivalent to the British Association of Plastic, Reconstructive and Aesthetic Surgeons (BAPRAS) and the Philippine Dental Association equivalent to our General Dental Council.

You can also expect surgeons to have international memberships such as with the International Society of Aesthetic Plastic Surgery (ISAPS) or the European Association of Plastic Surgeons (EURAPS). Ask whether those based in Europe are 'Board Certified'. Cosmetic surgeons trained in the US may be members of the American Society of Plastic Surgeons (ASPS).

Checking out the Clinic/hospital

Check to see that the proposed provider/country lists which professional regulatory bodies oversee its private clinics, and if not, ask. In the UK for example, the assessment of clinics is the responsibility of the Health and Safety Executive, the Healthcare Commission and local primary care organisations who conduct practice inspections.

Usually the Health Division of the country's government e.g. the Czech Ministry of Health oversees clinics along with the relevant country's Medical Council and/or associations. Ask for the name of the clinic/hospital where the surgery will be carried out, and find information online. Have a good read of the provider's web site which should have plenty of information about their clinics and services including details of the surgeon's qualifications/accreditation and what surgery they perform.

Some suggested questions include:

- Will the operation take place in a private hospital or at the doctor's clinic?
- Do they use an outpatient clinic or a hospital?
- Are they certified with the local and national health organisations?
- Do they have a crash cart (used in case of emergency)?
- How far is the clinic from an intensive care unit in case of emergency?
- What are the post operative infection rates?

Questions to ask the Surgeon or Dentist Overseas

There are many questions to ask the surgeon but the most important aspect is about safety, so grill the surgeon as much as you need until you feel reassured. If you don't understand something don't be afraid to say so - remember this is your body/teeth/life and what this surgeon does will remain with you for the rest of your life so make sure you have all of your questions answered. You are entitled to choose which surgeon performs your procedure, and not just be given whoever is available on that particular day.

Some suggested questions include:

- What professional memberships, training and qualifications do they hold? (Afterwards go to the relevant association's website to verify that their name is on the list)
- Have the surgeon and anaesthetist worked together before?

This is critical as they build up a relationship and can better monitor the patient's needs

- Will the anaesthetist perform a pre operative evaluation? And a post operative evaluation?
- Will the anaesthetist take into account the patient's wishes (provided it is safe to do so)?
- How much recovery time will the procedure entail?

- How long will you be hospitalised?
- How soon after the operation can you fly home?

Ask to see credentials and 'before and after' pictures.

As far as checking the rest of the medical team, remember that a good surgeon will only work with a good anaesthetist and in a good hospital/clinic - so the most important part is finding a good surgeon!

What Guarantee should you Expect?

Whether at home or abroad there are no guarantees regarding the result of any surgical or dental procedure, and this is especially true with plastic surgery where the results vary so much with each individual, and the perceived goal could be very different from the attainable goal.

However, the one guarantee a patient CAN ask for is that if a complication should arise, the surgeon or dentist will correct it without additional fees. Standards of legal protection for patients vary from country to country and once a provider is chosen, research the legal situation (you may wish to call the relevant country's embassy or consular office) and find out what protection you have as a visiting patient and use the web to research patient protection laws.

What to Check in the Document

Once you have decided on a provider or a broker ask for everything to be outlined in an agreement or contract which clearly describes the services provided to you at the agreed price. Check if there is anything you are not sure about and get someone else to read over the contract for you. Standards of legal protection for patients vary dramatically from country to country. One of the points that potential patients should check is the refund policy in case:

- o you change your mind once you arrive.
- o you have a pre existing medical condition that causes the surgery to be cancelled.
- o you can't get all the procedures yo u have paid for.

It is also important to clarify the clauses regarding follow-up care and what happens if anything goes wrong. This varies for someone having a hip replacement to someone having dental veneers but it is expected that the provider will stand by their patients and the work, and do whatever is necessary to make it right. Be sure to clarify this beforehand.

How to Compare Different Providers

The bottom line is to choose a provider/company/surgeon that you trust and feel most comfortable with. If the people you are dealing with seem unsympathetic or impatient with your questioning then take that as a sign and go elsewhere. As a paying customer, it is the patient's right to ask as much as they want to establish whether or not to go ahead with a procedure. Whether you are dealing with a provider directly or going through a broker be sure to address ALL of your questions and concerns beforehand, and to get a firm estimate/assessment of costs and scheduling - you won't want to deal with these issues after your procedure so be prepared, and don't be caught off guard. Every company has a different policy regarding the length of stay. The ideal length of stay will ensure that there are no complications and that the patient can come back home safely and without surprises. Choosing a company which offers holiday packages can be advantageous but should not distract from the main objective which is the surgery itself. Equally, hospitals or individual surgeons won't be as adept at organizing the logistics of travel or accommodation so if you're not a seasoned traveler it might be advisable to go through a broker who takes care of both.

Remember it is perfectly natural to have some anxiety before a major operation/dentistry/cosmetic procedure whether you are having it done in the UK, or abroad, but doing so in a foreign country will raise concerns about safety so ensure you do your research, ask questions and then ask some more until you feel confident that you are in good hands. If you are happy with the answers given, if you have done all the essential checking of the policy, verified their qualifications and credentials (as advised in this guide), feel comfortable about having the procedure in your chosen country and have done all your calculations so you know exactly what is involved in the cost and feel confident about the surgeon's abilities then you have probably found the right provider for your procedure. But if you have any doubts at all at this stage, voice them with the relevant people, or go to another provider.

What not to Do

- Go for cosmetic surgery or dentistry based only on pictures or email correspondence;
- Choose a country based solely on its tourist merits, without fully checking out the reputation of the surgeons, dentists, clinics or hospitals;
- Go ahead with a procedure if you're not fully comfortable or happy with what's happening, or with the surgeon who is going to do the procedure.
- Remember that you are entitled to change your mind at any time, even five minutes before the operation.

The Practicalities of going Abroad for Treatment

After the initial enquiry phone call or email has been made, and a formal quote for treatment received, the next step is the consultation process, to assess whether a patient is a good candidate for the procedure(s) requested. A consultation is also a good opportunity to learn about anything the surgeon requires you to do beforehand, such as lose weight or take certain vitamins to help the recovery process. With dentistry for example, it's normal that digital photos and x-rays are all the consultant sees until the patient arrives and pictures don't always show exactly what is going on, so a pre-consultation process with a local surgeon will not only help provide extra information to the surgeon abroad but make the patient's consultation more accurate.

Check that you have a valid passport. If it needs renewing pick up an application form from your local Post Office or apply online via the Passport Office. Check also whether you will need a visa to visit the country, how long this lasts and whether you can get it upon arrival or if it should be pre-arranged. Many providers/brokers will help and advise on visas and passport matters as part of their service. Make sure you take photocopies of your passport, visa and other documentation and keep them separate to your hand luggage and leave details of where you are going with someone at home. Don't forget to take the contact details of someone in the UK who can be contacted in case of emergency. Familiarise yourself with your chosen country's culture and customs. What are the local customs, religions and etiquette? Is it customary to tip, and if so, how much?

- It's a good idea to purchase some local currency in advance and take either traveler cheques or credit cards which can be used to withdraw money from local ATMs.
- Find out what clothing will be appropriate and make a list of some of the tourist attractions you might want to visit.
- You should also consider personal safety, check the Foreign Office website for any risks in the country you are visiting that you should be made aware of, and whether you can drink the local water or will need necessary vaccinations.
- With major operations plan recreational activities such as diving, surfing, hiking, safari tours, or taking a road trip before the procedure because time to relax and recover will be needed afterwards.

What to do if Something goes Wrong

All operations carry some risk and while it is hoped that all medical, dental, or cosmetic procedures will go to plan even with a smooth procedure it is wise to exercise some caution. Plan properly for the recovery period and anticipate any possible complications. Allow some flexibility to your schedule - just in case. Know what to expect - ask the doctor for detailed instructions and to explain what is normal and what is not for the days following the surgery. After an operation, complications can arise but immediate postoperative problems will be solved during a patient's stay in the hospital. Depending on the procedure a patient might do their own follow up care with their local GP so it is important:

(a) that you have a good and reliable GP in place and

(b) that you tell your GP that you are going abroad for treatment.

After cosmetic surgery procedures you are more likely to deal with UK medical specialists post op and some medical tourism providers include ongoing consultation with the UK specialist after your return to be sure that healing is successful and to ensure any concerns are addressed. It is important to clarify what is in place in terms of complications and risks of infection before going ahead with the procedure as policies vary between providers. If infections or other problems do occur once back in the UK you should get in touch with the surgeon, and follow their instructions. If you are really worried you should see your G.P. or go to the Accident and Emergency department of your local hospital if you can't get hold of your surgeon. If you are unhappy with your surgery or it has been badly performed talk to your surgeon immediately to seek a resolution.

Medical Tourism and the Cosmetic Surgery Scene in the Philippines

More and more people from all over the world are traveling to other countries not only as tourists who come for sightseeing and shopping but also to get medical, dental, and surgical services from hospitals and other health destinations. Medical tourism is a rapidly growing industry with countries like Cuba, Costa Rica, Hungary, India, Israel, Jordan, Lithuania, Malaysia, South Africa and Thailand actively promoting it. The Philippines is also fast becoming a favored destination for patients seeking quality medical care at very affordable prices. The high costs of healthcare in industrialized countries, the improved standards in foreign countries and the lower costs of air travel have made medical tourism a popular trend. In the Philippines, both local and foreign patients who otherwise couldn't afford medical procedures such as plastic surgery benefit from the highly favorable exchange rate. The cost savings are significant. For example, if the average surgeon's fee for eyelid surgery in the U.S. is $2,500, in the Philippines, a qualified surgeon will charge only $600 to $1,500. For liposuction, surgeon's fees in the U.S. average $2,000 per area. In the Philippines, it is around $800 for the first area and $500 for succeeding areas. Anesthesiologist's fees and facility costs are also much lower.

Lower overhead costs and professional fees makes it possible for surgeons to perform these surgeries at a fraction of the cost of the same procedures in the United States, U.K. and other countries, without sacrificing quality of care. The Philippines' medical services can rival the best in the world and a significant number of foreigners are choosing to undergo their cosmetic plastic surgery procedures such as liposuction, breast augmentation, rhinoplasty, face lift, tummy tuck and blepharoplasty at local hospitals and out-patient surgeries. Patients also usually appreciate the added benefit that they are away from their surroundings during the recuperation period, with no friends and family to see them when looking less than their best after the operation. Whether patients are having cosmetic surgery abroad or in their home country, choosing the right surgeon is the single most important decision they will make.

In the Philippines, there are many qualified and well-trained doctors who have had formal training in plastic and reconstructive surgery, have acquired their postgraduate or fellowship training from well-known institutions in the U.S.A. and have been mentored by leading plastic surgeons. To enhance their expertise, they regularly attend various seminars worldwide, where new techniques in plastic and cosmetic surgery are introduced.

The greater acceptance and growth of cosmetic surgery among the general public has encouraged many Filipino doctors to perform cosmetic plastic surgery. However, not all of them have trained as plastic surgeons. Once doctors get their medical degrees, they may practice any specialty, even if they have not completed advanced training in the field they have chosen. And so, a doctor who performs cosmetic plastic surgery is not necessarily trained as a plastic surgeon. To ensure best results, patients should choose an authentic plastic surgeon with the training and experience that is essential for the success of their surgery. When foreign patients choose to have their elective cosmetic surgeries done by qualified plastic surgeons in Philippines, they get exceptional value for the latest techniques in cosmetic plastic surgery. They combine having a vacation in a beautiful tropical country with affordable, quality elective plastic surgery.

Guidelines for Cosmetic Surgery Tourism

A growing number of medical tourists are availing of cosmetic surgery when they go on vacation to the Philippines. Many of them are "balikbayan" Filipino immigrants or overseas workers visiting relatives and friends. They often regard cosmetic surgery as a last-minute item on their shopping list, something which can be done during the last few days of their vacation. If a patient is seriously considering cosmetic surgery, the vacation should be planned such that enough time is allotted for the following: pre-operative consultation (1 day), pre-operative laboratory work-up (1 day), actual surgery date (1 day) and time for post-operative recovery (1 to 2 weeks). The American Society of Plastic Surgeons (ASPS) has issued an advisory that before flying, a patient should wait for five to seven days after body procedures such as liposuction and breast augmentation, and seven to 10 days after cosmetic procedures of the face including facelifts, eyelid surgery, nose jobs, and laser treatments. If a patient has limited vacation time, having the pre-operative laboratory work up (blood tests, electrocardiogram, and chest x-ray) done prior to their vacation will facilitate scheduling of the surgery. A patient with medical insurance coverage may be entitled to a laboratory work up as part of their annual physical examination package.

Patients with risk factors such as diabetes or cardiovascular disease will also need to consult their primary care doctor, HMO physician, cardiologist, or internist, and must secure a written clearance that they are physically fit to undergo the contemplated cosmetic surgery procedure. Once all these necessary pre-operative precautions are undertaken, the next step is to choose a qualified plastic surgeon. Patients will be taking unnecessary risks if they choose unqualified doctors to do their cosmetic surgery. Patients should also make sure that their operation will be performed in a facility that is well-equipped.

In recent years, it has been noted by the international media that the high cost of cosmetic surgery in the U.S.A., Europe and Australia has resulted in the price-driven phenomenon known as cosmetic surgery tourism. Since medical insurance does not cover the cost of cosmetic surgery and patients have to pay out-of-pocket, price has become a major factor in promoting cosmetic surgery tourism. Thus patients from First World countries have chosen the alternative of flying to countries where cosmetic surgery is more affordable. The growth of cosmetic surgery tourism is a sign of international recognition of the capabilities of plastic surgeons who have chosen to live and work in "Second or Third World" countries.

A cursory Internet search will show entire cosmetic surgery "vacation packages" that cost less than single cosmetic surgery procedures done in the U.S.A. Many companies are offering cosmetic surgery vacation packages which generally include hospital, hotel or resort accommodations together with the cosmetic surgery. However, it must be pointed out that vacation-related activities should be avoided after surgery. Patients should avoid sun exposure, walking tours, bus tours, alcohol-intake, smoking or exposure to second-hand smoke, exercise, and water activities (swimming, snorkeling, scuba diving, water skiing, jet-skiing, parasailing, etc.). To help ensure optimal results and to limit risks and complications, patients should not treat cosmetic surgery lightly and must observe all the necessary precautions during both pre-operative and post-operative periods.

Cosmetic Surgery Today

Cosmetic or aesthetic surgery is a very popular subject these days. Make a search on the internet for cosmetic or plastic surgery and you will get millions of results - web sites of plastic surgeons of different nationalities, various procedures available, advice for cheap plastic surgery, before and after photos, celebrity patients, clinics and surgery travel packages for various countries, news from around the world, and more.

There is an increasing number of individuals from all walks of life who undergo cosmetic surgery each year. What is cosmetic surgery and why are so many people interested in it? Cosmetic surgery is a highly sophisticated surgical specialty that is dedicated not only to the return of the face and body to normal but to improvements that actually surpass the normal. Well, is it simply that more people nowadays want to "surpass the normal" or be above average in appearance than before? Not really. Several factors are responsible for the boom in cosmetic surgery today. Several factors such as the media are responsible for the boom in cosmetic surgery today.

Destination Medical Tourism Philippines

Philippine Health Tourism Programme (PHTP) aims to target both the wellness/spa and medical tourist markets. Tourism Secretary Roberto Pagdanganan, said that health holidays are significantly growing outside Europe and in other parts of the world - "If the growth of health resorts in Asia, including the Philippines, is anything to go by, there would seem to be a huge potential to develop health tourism as a great come-on since health and wellness using traditional healing methods, such as massage, healing and herbs is very much part of the Asian culture."

Under the Philippine Health Tourism Program (PHTP), DOT and its partner agencies such as the Department of Health-Philippine Institute of Traditional and Alternative Health Care (DOH-PITAHC) and the Department of Energy (DOE) are jointly offering cost-effective medical treatments combined with special itineraries that will showcase some of the best tourist attractions the country could offer. The new program will be offered to tourists whose main purpose for visiting the Philippines is to undergo "minimally invasive medical procedures and treatments." Specially-designed tours integrated with the medical programs by accredited hospitals and healthcare establishments will then be offered to suit the needs of these identified market segment.

Philippines is one of the few countries in Asia to offer such specialized medical or health tour offerings, with only Thailand,

Malaysia, Singapore and India as competitors. The DOT, DOH-PITAHC and DOE have already come up with rules and regulations for the accreditation of health establishments, wellness centers and hospitals in the country, using DOT's standards for hotels as the benchmark.

Currently, only St. Luke's Medical Center remains the only hospital that has met these standards. Hospitals such as the Asian Hospital in Alabang, Capitol Medical Center in Quezon City and Medical City in Mandaluyong City are gearing up to offer world class facilities. Surgeons in the Philippines, routinely perform kidney transplants and complicated cardiac procedures.

The country's bid was also reinforced during the state visit of President Gloria Macapagal-Arroyo in Bahrain last December when the Bahraini government expressed interest to send medical tourists to the Philippines.

Now underway are a Medical Tourism Forum and modules for the implementation of a "Mabuhay Host Training Program" for healthcare frontliners of accredited hospitals, all to strengthen the country's readiness as a health vacation destination. The DOT is also spearheading the establishment of the Spa Philippines Association (SPA), an organization to be composed of accredited firms and individuals who are directly or indirectly engaged in the spa business.

The SPA, which will be DOT's ally in promoting the Philippines as a spa holiday destination in Asia, aims to uphold the standards and ethics of the Philippine spa industry and strive towards its professionaliszation, ensure the highest standards of services and facilities for clients, and develop a unique branding or image for the Philippine spa industry.

One of the most active participants in the DOT's Philippine Health Tourism Program, The Farm at San Benito-Hippocrates Health Resort of Asia, a world-class alternative medical resort in Lipa City Batangas, holds healthful activities for the whole family.

Called "Family Week at the Farm," this series of activities is part of the health resort's commitment to the DOT to help in promoting the country as a health vacation destination in

Asia. Activities which a family will surely enjoy include kite flying, arts and crafts, massage lessons for kids, face painting, yoga, conscious walking exercise, swimming, seed planting, healthy food preparation, etc. The Farm includes a fully integrated medical facility specializing in alternative preventive health and natural healing.

Philippine Medical Tourism:Cosmetic Surgery in the Philippines

The Philippines is now on its way to becoming a top destination for medical tourism worldwide. Philippine cosmetic plastic surgery is one of the more popular services sought after. Cosmetic surgery has been on an upward trend worldwide especially with the constant and continuous development of surgical and non surgical techniques in recent years... from laser resurfacings to thread lifts...from endoscopic lift surgeries to minimally invasive rejuvenating techniques...

Unfortunately these relatively new and popular elective procedures together with the traditional and effective surgeries are not always accessible and affordable even to those living in developed countries as the United States, United Kingdom, Australia, countries in Europe and parts of Asia. Medical and health services there in general have always been expensive. Cost of course has always been a significant factor and important consideration among many other things for the potential patient...it is after all something universal...The good news though is that certain select countries such as Mexico, Brazil, India, Singapore, Malaysia, Thailand and the Philippines just to name a few, have taken notice and have taken advantage of this dilemma by offering these surgeries at very affordable rates to interested patients outside their territories.

The significant price differential between medical and surgical costs between these developed countries and the Philippines in particular have made patients abroad take a second look at this attractive option. Who won't be amazed with getting a surgery package cost of about a third to a quarter of the price found in most developed countries with just the same results?

Medical tourism in the Philippines has actually been silently ongoing for decades now however it has only been recently wherein the Department of Tourism has actually emphasized and strongly encouraged the Medical profession to join the band wagon. In Asia, Thailand still leads the way in organized and systematic channeling of medical tourism services particularly in cosmetic plastic surgery.

The Philippines is rapidly catching up though and is steadily getting a bigger share of the pie. In 2006, the Department of Health in cooperation with the Department of Tourism came up with the Philippine Medical Tourism Program (PMTP) which is a multisectoral program with the ultimate goal of making the Philippines the leading and foremost destination for wellness and medical care in Asia.

Aggressive local and overseas promotion and an improving tourism infrastructure is a priority of the Philippine government and has brought a significant boost in medical tourism in the country. Initially driven and encouraged by very competitive rates and costs of surgery in this part of the world, patients are now flying in with the desire of having surgery and rejuvenation with the added bonus of seeing and experiencing the best places these islands can offer.

Tagaytay, Batangas, Boracay, Cebu, Palawan, and Davao are just some of the more popular tourist destinations which have caught the eye of our foreign visitors and "balikbayans". However, sometimes unknowingly, providing much leverage in the development of this relatively new industry is actually and simply the inherent qualities of being a Filipino. The Filipino physician and support staff are typically compassionate, caring, friendly and hospitable. This not only helps in making a foreign patient comfortable and relaxed but also eventually makes his trip and surgery a very pleasant experience. Aside from being generally fluent in the English language, the Filipino medical work force is competitive and of high standards as compared to their Asian neighbors.

Therefore when patients coming from abroad do decide to have elective cosmetic plastic surgeries here in the country, more often than not they get excellent value for their money.

Medical and surgical expertise, world class facilities and island destinations, mastery of English, and the typical Filipino, all contribute to the Philippines rise to global competitiveness in medical tourism.

Simply put and everything said nothing beats a combined quality and affordable surgery in the setting of a tropical paradise for leisure and recuperation. Medical tourism is the practice of traveling to another country in order to receive medical enhancement, be it heart surgery, breast implants, a hip replacement, or dental work. Depending on the location and procedure, a medical vacation can wind up costing a mere fraction of what you would pay at home.

Even when you factor in air fare, hotels, travel insurance, car rental, shopping, and dining, many medical vacations are substantially more affordable than domestic health care. For example, a heart valve operation that might require you to pay $100,000 in the States could cost well under $10,000 in a country like India where lower labor costs help drive down the price considerably. The same is true in popular medical tourism destinations like Mexico, Thailand, and Hungary.

MEDICAL TOURISM TODAY

Throughout much of recorded history, traveling for curative reasons was restricted either to the wealthy or to the truly desperate. But in today's flattening global economy, the physical, economic, and cultural borders that once separated nations from one another are wearing away as international travel, mass communication, and more lenient trade policies make it possible for those with modest means to enjoy the benefits of world-class health care treatments.

These advancements translate into a smorgasbord of options for patients who find it difficult or impossible to access affordable health care in their own countries. Today, Americans, failed by grossly inflated health care costs flock to hospitals in countries like Thailand for sophisticated procedures at a fraction of the price. In countries like England, where socialized medicine is the norm, long wait times and insufficient health care personnel have helped produce a steady stream of medical tourists to countries like India where a highly evolved education system produces thousands of qualified doctors and nurses (many of whom also study in the West). Low labor costs, quality medical schools, and heavy investing are helping to transform many parts of the developing world into medical tourism hotspots that show no sign of stopping.

While affordability and time are still the main reasons why patients trudge across borders for treatment, it can't be denied that quality of care is a major factor as well. In fact, it's sometimes better than what you would expect from unmotivated and sluggish primary health care centers back home. Most countries vying for a slice of the multi-billion dollar medical tourism pie have expanded their offerings, invested heavily in medical infrastructure, and begun advertising aggressively.

4

Thailand Medical Tourism

If foreigners have a medical problems while in Thailand, they invariably seem to end up in one of a few hospitals that have a good reputation, and are well known to cater to foreign patients. Bumrungrad Hospital (Sukhumvit soi 1) seems to be most popular among residents in the Sukhumvit area.

However Bangkok General Hospital and its affiliates Samitivej Hospital (Sukhumvit Soi 49) and Bangkok Nursing Home Hospital (Convent Road, off Silom Road), are also very popular. The last 4 or 5 years the above mentioned hospitals have been actively (together with a general promotional attitude by the authorities) seeking medical tourists to visit Thailand. Amazingly up to 60% of patients at Bumrungrad Hospital and up to 40 % of patients at Samitivej Hospital are foreigners. We do not think that Thai patients are not accepted in these hospitals. It just so happens that while foreigners may consider the hospitals cheaper than in their home countries, for most Thais they are simply to expensive to consider.

Samitivej Hospital (part of the Bangkok General Hospital Group) is upmarket and is one of the health care providers for medical tourists in Thailand. It is located about 3 km into soi 49, Sukhumvit Road. The Kasikorn Research Centre reported that 1.28 million expatriates visited Thai Hospitals in 2005, generating revenue for these hospitals of around 33 billion baht. On average, this means each foreign patient paid 25,800 baht for services provided. The average reflects most likely more expensive procedures such as major surgery, and a whole lot of out patient clinic visits. We assume that this includes also a lot of 'annual check-ups'. Bumrungrad Hospital is much in the news media. It has been covered on U.S. television stations, and also in international magazines. Also the local English press seems to have an article about the hospital every few weeks. Surely, the public relations office at the hospital is doing a superb job.

An article in Newsweek (October 2006) reveals that Bumrungrad hospital treated 400,000 foreign patients in 2005. This number is astounding and must be (not clearly stated in the article) referring to total hospital visits rather than total number of patients treated. Furthermore, the hospital is in the process of finishing a new 18-story outpatient center, which will increase the hospital's outpatient capacity to 6,000 patients per day.

Medical tourism will certainly generate further income for the hospitals involved and for Thailand in general. Thailand assets as a center for medical care for foreigners are multiple. The standard of treatment and technology is high (see : 64-Slice Computer Tomography Scanner ; Adult Stem Cell Treatment in Thailand).

The prices are mostly lower than in other countries who provide similar quality and technology. The hospital environment in Thailand is clearly more hospitable. It is fair to say that all the hospitals mentioned above, also look good, are mostly new, and give a favorable impression as soon as you enter them.

The tourism infrastructure is well developed (provided you are not so sick that you can not really enjoy sightseeing). Income from medical tourism to Thailand is projected to increase in the following years. It has to be recognized that 33 billion baht of income (about 850 million US dollar) is only a small proportion of the total income generated by tourism. Development of Thailand as a medical hub for patients from the United States, Europe, the surrounding countries, and the Middle East, also raises questions.

Possibly the most important is : does this all affect the medical care for the Thai population itself? As stated above, most Thai patients can not afford to go to private hospitals. So where to they go to? Over the last few years the Thai Government has developed the so-called '30 baht scheme'. This is a universal healtcare programme whereby everybody get treatment at public hospitals for a standard fee per visit of only just 30 baht. Basically this amounts to free health care.

The hospitals who participate in the scheme, get a lump sum per patient registered. We think at present it amounts to somewhat less than 2,000 baht per patient. It has to be recognized as a major achievement, since before that there hardly was any proper healtcare available for the poorer (that is the larger) part of the population. However, you have to use your own imagination as to whether the Thai population benefiting from this scheme, will receive the same standard of treatment, as the foreigners who are treated at private hospitals.

Another issue is as to where physicians will prefer to work? There is a long standing problem of a lack of medical specialists in certain provinces of Thailand. While the training of just one doctor takes quite a lot of government resources, it does not follow that the doctors trained feel obliged to go and work in some remote area.

Furthermore, we are quite certain that salaries paid by physicians working at private hospitals are higher. So there will be a tendency for highly specialized doctors to work in private hospitals at the expense of the care provided in public hospitals for the general public. While spas and meditation are designed to help prevent health problems, a huge business is being generated amongst those who already nave problems, and need treatment. Many Thai hospitals and medical centers, which have recently been listed on The Stock Exchange of Thailand to raise funds for investment in equipment and construction, see a formidable revenue stream in attracting clients for medical check-ups. At present, the cost of getting a medical check-up in Thailand is a fraction of what it costs in more developed countries. Language problems notwithstanding, a number of major Thai hospitals have learned the ropes of the travel business and are marketing themselves to also regular participants at international trade shows, like

ITB in Berlin and the Arabian Travel Mart. At Thailand 's more than 400 private hospitals, standards are high and costs are extremely competitive. Little surprise then that large numbers of visitors decide to undergo surgery in the Kingdom as part of their stay. Whether you are after plastic surgery, lasik eye treatment or major heart surgery, you can rely on round the-clock, quality service in Bangkok and the min provincial cities and tourist centers, Seeking care on holiday is a trouble-free experience.

Doctors and specialists can swiftly obtain patient records by satellite. Hospitals employ staff fluent in English and who have overseas training. Demand for their services from he middle East has also led to the hiring of Arabic-speaking personnel. Indeed, the whole business of linkage between the hospitals and the travel industry took a step forward when Thai Airways International (THAI) began packaging medical check-ups as part of its Royal Orchid Holidays programme.

HIGH STANDARD OF MEDICAL SERVICES

Thai hospital is renowned around the world, and is a fact of which the Thais are very proud. This asset also plays vital part in the private health services in which the quality and the standard are exceptionally high. With the country gearing towards long-stay health lifestyle tourism, medical services play an important part as well. At present, Thailand has more than 400 private hospitals scattered throughout the kingdom. Most of the hospitals are staffed with overseas-trained doctors and a specialist who can ensure that communication is no barrier.

There are fast mobile service including helicopter and aircraft, and patients' records can be swiftly obtained via the internet. Visitor who choose to long-stay in Thailand can rest assured that Thailand's private hospitals are of very high standard while the fees are surprising low compared to those on the West. Foreign expatriates, executives of international corporations and embassy staff will all attest to the excellence of hospital treatment here and to its comparatively low cost. Whether you are contemplating a check-up pr a major medical professional procedure, you will enjoy prompt attention, immaculate comfort, highly profession staff, and friendly faces.

In recent years, "medical tourism" has become the new buzzword for the development of Thailand's tourism industry. What this means is encouraging people to come to Thailand, have a little elective surgery, and then recuperate on some nice beach.

The idea is not as crazy as it may sound. Some of Thailand's private hospitals are capable of world class healthcare, accredited according some of the toughest standards around. While they might be expensive for many Thais, these hospitals are still able to offer a high standard of care for far less than a hospital stay in most western countries will cost. We're not talking about critical care, such as transplants. Medical Tourism is targeted at elective and non-emergency treatments, such as cosmetic surgery or hip replacements. Such are the cost savings that some insurance companies will not only cover the costs of treatment, but some of the travel costs as well, to have work done in Thailand. Thailand's low cost health care is not limited to medical treatment. Thanks to tight government price controls, most medicines cost far less than they do in western countries.

Thai Hospitals: Here's a short list of hospitals that specialize in treating foreigners. They all have staff who speak English, as well as many other languages. All of the institutions below are based in Bangkok, although some have branches in other parts of the country.

Bumrungrad International Hospital : Perhaps the most advanced and internationalized of Thailand's private hospital. Coming here can seem like a visit to a five star hotel and the United Nations all in one. Although comparatively expensive for Thais, the hospital gets many foreign visitors in search of high quality health care at reasonable cost. The web site provides an overview of the hospital's services, and the ability to make appointments online.

Bangkok General Hospital : A good general medicine hospital. The web site is available in many languages. The main services for foreign visitors are cosmetic surgery. The hospital can arrange for a variety of treatments as part of your holiday.

Samitivej Hospital : Samitivej is one of Bangkok's most respected hospitals. Its main claim to fame is the "baby friendly" natal facilities. It's probably unlikely that you would want to travel to Thailand to have your baby, but the hospital has several other services to offer as well, including extensive children's healthcare departments.

St. Carlos Hospital : This small hospital has combined traditional medicine with a full fledged spa to provide a complete range of health and beauty treatments, from cosmetic surgery to detoxifying body treatments.

Rutnin Eye Hospital : Rutnin is perhaps Bangkok's largest eye hospital, with a full range of services such as lasik corrections. Sort of a medical travel planner, providing a concierge type service to help you plan your trip to Bangkok for cosmetic surgery or other medical procedures. They can help you to plan your trip, select doctors and facilities, and schedule your appointments or procedures before you arrive.

5

A Broad Horizon

Tourism is the act of travel for predominantly recreational or leisure purposes, and also refers to the provision of services in support of this act. According to the World Tourism Organization, tourists are people who "travel to and stay in places outside their usual environment for not more than one consecutive year for leisure, business and other purposes not related to the exercise of an activity remunerated from within the place visited". Tourism, however long its incident duration, has become an extremely popular, global activity. In 2004, there were over 763 million international tourist arrivals.

As a service industry, tourism has numerous tangible and intangible elements. Major tangible elements include transportation, accommodation, and other components of a hospitality industry. Major intangible elements relate to the purpose or motivation for becoming a tourist, such as rest, relaxation, the opportunity to meet new people and experience other cultures, or simply to do something different and have an adventure. Tourism is vital for many countries, due to the income generated by the consumption of goods and services by tourists, the taxes levied on businesses in the tourism industry, and the opportunity for employment and economic advancement by working in the industry.

For these reasons NGOs and government agencies may sometimes promote a specific region as a tourist destination, and support the development of a tourism industry in that area. The contemporary phenomenon of mass tourism may sometimes result in overdevelopment, however alternative forms of tourism such as ecotourism seek to avoid such outcomes by pursuing tourism in a sustainable way. The terms tourism and travel are sometimes used interchangeably. In this context travel has a similar definition to tourism, but implies a more purposeful journey. The terms tourism and tourist are sometimes used pejoratively to imply a shallow interest in the cultures or locations visited by tourists.

DEFINITION, CLASSIFICATION AND PREREQUISITES

General Definition

One of the earliest definitions of tourism was provided by the Austrian economist Hermann Von Schullard in 1910, who defined it as, "sum total of operators, mainly of an economic nature, which directly relate to the entry, stay and movement of foreigners inside and outside a certain country, city or a region."

Hunziker and Krapf, in 1941, defined tourism as "the sum of the phenomena and relationships arising from the travel and stay of non-residents, in so far as they do not lead to permanent residence and are not connected with any earning activity."

In 1976 Tourism Society of England defined it as "Tourism is the temporary, short-term movement of people to destination outside the places where they normally live and work and their activities during the stay at each destination. It includes movements for all purposes."

In 1981 International Association of Scientific Experts in Tourism defined Tourism in terms of particular activities selected by choice and undertaken outside the home environment.

United Nations Definition

United Nations classified 3 forms of tourism in 1994 in its Recommendations on Tourism Statistics as follows:

1. Domestic tourism, involving residents of the given country traveling only within this country;
2. Inbound tourism, involving non-residents traveling in the given country;

3. Outbound tourism, involving residents traveling in another country.

UN also derived different categories of tourism by combining the 3 basic forms of tourism:

1. Internal tourism, which comprises domestic tourism and inbound tourism;
2. National tourism, which comprises domestic tourism and outbound tourism;
3. International tourism, which consists of inbound tourism and outbound tourism.

New Definition

Intrabound tourism is a new academic terminology coined by the Korea tourism organization and widely accepted in Korea. Intrabound tourism differs from 'domestic tourism' in that the former is more dynamic and comprehensive, encompassing policy-making and implementation of national tourism policies in consideration of the tourism ecosystem consisting of inbound, outbound and intrabound tourism. Entering into 21st century, the tourism industry has undergone a paradigm shift form the promotion of inbound tourism to the promotion of intrabound tourism since many countries are experiencing a tough competition for inbound tourists. Also realizing that it is impossible to advance the inbound tourism in the absence of active intrabound tourism, national policy makers have shifted their policy priority onto the promotion of intrabound tourism such as the promotion of local tourism to contribute to the local economy.

Examples of such policies are "See America," "Getting Going Canada," and "See Korea Campaign". Taking a Korean case as an example, Korea Tourism Organization has recently launched a nation-wide campaign to promote introbound tourism, named "Guseok Guseok, literally meaning corner to corner..

PREREQUISITES OF TOURISM

Before people are able to experience tourism they usually need at least:

1. disposable income, i.e. money to spend on non-essentials
2. leisure time
3. tourism infrastructure, such as transport and accommodation

Individually, sufficient health is also a condition, and of course the inclination to travel. Furthermore, in some countries there are legal restrictions on travelling, especially abroad. Certain states with strong governmental control over the lives of citizens (notably established Communist states) may restrict foreign travel only to trustworthy citizens. The United States prohibits its citizens from traveling to some countries, for example, Cuba.

HISTORY

Wealthy people have always travelled to distant parts of the world to see great buildings or other works of art, to learn new languages, to experience new cultures, or to taste new cuisine. As long ago as the time of the Roman Republic places such as Baiae were popular coastal resorts for the rich. The terms tourist and tourism were first used as official terms in 1937 by the League of Nations. Tourism was defined as people travelling abroad for periods of over 24 hours.

TYPES OF TOURISM

Health Tourism and Leisure Travel

The history of European tourism can perhaps be said to originate with the medieval pilgrimage. Although undertaken primarily for religious reasons, the pilgrims in the Canterbury Tales quite clearly saw the experience as a kind of holiday (the term itself being derived from the 'holy day' and its associated leisure activities).

Pilgrimages created a variety of tourist aspects that still exist-bringing back souvenirs, obtaining credit with foreign banks (in medieval times utilising international networks established by Jews and Lombards), and making use of space available on existing forms of transport (such as the use of medieval English wine ships bound for Vigo by pilgrims to

Santiago De Compostela). Pilgrimages are still important in modern tourism-such as to Lourdes or Knock in Ireland. But there are modern equivalents-Graceland and the grave of Jim Morrison in Père Lachaise Cemetery.

During the seventeenth century, it became fashionable in England to undertake a Grand Tour. The sons of the nobility and gentry were sent upon an extended tour of Europe as an educational experience. The eighteenth century was the golden age of the Grand Tour, and many of the fashionable visitors were painted at Rome by Pompeo Batoni. A modern equivalent of the Grand Tour is the phenomenon of the backpacker, although cultural holidays, such as those offered by Swann-Hellenic, are also important.

Health tourism has always existed, but it was not until the eighteenth century that it became important. In England, it was associated with spas, places with supposedly health-giving mineral waters, treating diseases from gout to liver disorders and bronchitis. Bath was the most fashionable resort, but Buxton, Harrogate, and Tunbridge Wells, amongst others, also flourished. Of course, people visited these places for the balls and other entertainments, just as much as 'the waters'. Continental Spas such as Karlsbad attracted many fashionable travellers by the nineteenth century.

It could be argued that Britain was the home of the seaside holiday. In travelling to the coast, the population was following in the steps of Royalty. King George III made regular visits to Weymouth when in poor health. At the time, a number of doctors argued the benefits of bathing in sea water, and sea bathing as a widespread practice was popularised by the Prince Regent (later George IV), who frequented Brighton for this purpose.

Leisure travel was associated with the industrialization of United Kingdom-the first European country to promote leisure time to the increasing industrial population. Initially, this applied to the owners of the machinery of production, the economic oligarchy, the factory owners, and the traders. These comprised the new middle class. Cox & Kings were the first official travel company to be formed in 1758. Later, the working class could take advantage of leisure time. The British origin of this new industry is reflected in many place names. At Nice, one of the first and best-established holiday resorts on the French Riviera, the long esplanade along the seafront is known to this day as the Promenade des Anglais; in many other historic resorts in continental Europe, old well-established palace hotels have names like the Hotel Bristol, the Hotel Carlton or the Hotel Majestic-reflecting the dominance of English customers.

Winter Tourism

Winter sports were largely invented by the British leisured classes, initially at the Swiss village of Zermatt (Valais), and St Moritz in 1864. The first packaged winter sports holidays took place in 1902 at Adelboden, Switzerland. Winter sports were a natural answer for a leisured class looking for amusement during the coldest season.

Organized sport was well established in Britain before it reached other countries. The vocabulary of sport bears witness to this: rugby, football, and boxing all originated in Britain, and even tennis, originally a French sport, was formalized and codified by the British, who hosted the first national championship in the nineteenth century, at Wimbledon.

The Fun Ski & Snow Festival, which has been organized annually by Korea tourism organization since 1998 and participated by about 10,000 tourists from Asia, is one of the most successful winter tourism products in Asia.

The festival provides a variety of events such as ski and sled competitions, ski and snow board lessons, performances and recreational activities. Majority of the event participants are foreign visitors who come from countries with a warm climate that have no snow. The event offers them opportunities to enjoy winter and winter sports in Korea.

In addition, southern South American countries making up the Patagonia region in Chile and Argentina attract thousands of tourists every year. Skiing is extremely popular in the mountanous areas.

Mass Travel

Mass travel could only develop with two crucial features:

1. improvements in technology allowed the transport of large numbers of people in a short space of time to places of leisure interest, and
2. greater numbers of people began to enjoy the benefits of leisure time.

The pioneer of modern mass tourism was Thomas Cook who, on 5 July 1841, organized the first package tour in history. He arranged for the rail company to charge one shilling per person for a group of 570 temperance campaigners from Leicester to a rally in Loughborough, eleven miles away. Cook was paid a share of the fares actually charged to the passengers, as the railway tickets, being legal contracts between company and passenger, could not have been issued at his own price. There had been railway excursions before, but this one included entrance to an entertainment held in private grounds, rail tickets and food for the train journey. Cook immediately saw the potential of a convenient 'off the peg' holiday product in which everything was included in one cost. He organised packages inclusive of accommodation for the Great Exhibition, and afterwards pioneered package holidays in both Britain (particularly in Scotland) and on the European continent (where Paris and the Alps were the most popular destinations).

He was soon followed by others (the Polytechnic Touring Association, Dean and Dawson etc.), with the result that the tourist industry developed rapidly in late Victorian Britain. Initially it was supported by the growing middle classes, who had time off from their work, and who could afford the luxury of travel and possibly even staying for periods of time in boarding houses.

The Bank Holidays Act 1871 introduced a statutory right for workers to take holidays, even if they were not paid at the time. By the last quarter of the nineteenth century, the tradition of the working class holiday had become firmly established in Britain. These were largely focussed upon the seaside resorts. The spread of the railway network in the nineteenth century resulted in the growth of Britain's seaside towns by bringing them within easy distance of Britain's urban centres.

Blackpool was created by the construction of a line to Fleetwood, and some resorts were promoted by the railway companies themselves-Morecambe by the Midland Railway and Cleethorpes by the Great Central Railway. Other resorts included Scarborough in Yorkshire, servicing Leeds and Bradford; Weston-super-Mare in Somerset, catering for the inhabitants of Bristol; and Skegness, patronised by the residents of the industrial East Midlands. The cockneys of London flocked to Southend-on-Sea, mainly by Thames Steamer, and the South Coast resorts such as Broadstairs, Brighton, and Eastbourne were only a train ride away, with others further afield such as Bournemouth, Bognor Regis and Weymouth.

For a century, domestic tourism was the norm, with foreign travel being reserved for the rich or the culturally curious. A number of inland destinations, such as the English Lake District, and Snowdonia appealed to those who liked the countryside and fine scenery.

The holiday camp began to appear in the 1930s, but this phenomenon really expanded in the post-war period. Butlins and Pontins set this trend, but their popularity waned with the rise of overseas package tours and the increasing comforts to which visitors became accustomed at home. Towards the end of the 20th century this market has been revived by the upmarket inland resorts of Dutch company Center Parcs.

Cox & Co, the forebear of Cox & Kings were in existence from 1758 largely entwined with the travel arrangements for the British Army serving around the Empire. While acting as 'agents' for various regiments, they organised the payment, provision, clothing and travel arrangements for members of the armed forces. In the 19th century their network of offices contained a banking and also travel department. The company became heavily involved with affairs in India and its Shipping Agency had offices in France and the Middle East.

Other phenomena that helped develop the travel industry were paid holidays:

- 1.5 million manual workers in Britain had paid holidays by 1925
- 11 million by 1939 (30% of the population in families with paid holidays)

INTERNATIONAL MASS TOURISM

Increasing speed on railways meant that the tourist industry could develop internationally.

To this may be added the development of sea travel. By 1901, the number of people crossing the English Channel from England to France or Belgium had passed 0.5 million per year. Shipping companies were anxious to fill cabin space that was under utilised. For example, P&O found that the majority of their passengers for India and the Far East joined the ship at Marseilles. Consequently, they marketed holidays based upon sea trips from London to Lisbon and Gibraltar. Other companies diverted their older ships to operate cruises in the summer months.

However, the real age of international mass travel began with the growth of air travel after World War Two. In the immediate post-war period, there was a surplus of transport aircraft, such as the popular and reliable Douglas Dakota, and a number of ex military pilots ready to fly them. They were available for charter flights, and tour operators began to use them for European destinations, such as Paris and Ostend.

Vladimir Raitz pioneered modern package tourism when on 20 May 1950 his recently founded company, Horizon, provided arrangements for a two-week holiday in Corsica. For an all inclusive price of £32.10s.-, holiday makers could sleep under canvas, sample local wines and eat a meal containing meat twice a day-this was especially attractive due to the continuing austerity measures in post-war United Kingdom. Within ten years, his company had started mass tourism to Palma (1952), Lourdes (1953), Costa Brava (1954), Sardinia (1954), Minorca (1955), Porto (1956), Costa Blanca (1957) and Costa del Sol (1959). However it was with cheap air travel in combination with the package tour that international mass tourism developed. The postwar introduction of an international system of airline regulation was another important factor. The bilateral agreements at the heart of the system fixed seat prices, and airlines could not fill blocks of empty seats on underused flights by discounting. But if they were purchased by a tour operator and hidden within the price of an inclusive holiday package, it would be difficult to prove that discounting had taken place-even though it was obvious that it had! This was the origin of the modern mass package tour.

These developments coincided with a significant increase in the standard of living in Britain. At the end of the 1950s, Harold Macmillan could say "you've never had it so good." Another significant development also happened at the end of this decade. The devaluation of the Spanish peseta made Spain appear a particularly attractive destination. The cheapness of the cost of living attracted increasing numbers of visitors.

Mass package tourism has at times been an exploitative process, in which tour operators in a country with a high standard of living make use of development opportunities and low operating costs in a country with a lower standard of living. However, as witness the development of many tourist areas in previously poor parts of the world, and the concomitant rise in standards of living, when there is equality of bargaining power, both parties can gain economic benefits from this arrangement.

Spain and the Balearic Islands became major tourist destinations, and development probably peaked in the 1980s. At the same time, British tour operators developed the Algarve in Portugal. The continuing search for new, cheaper, destinations spread mass tourism to the Greek Islands, Italy, Tunisia, Morocco, parts of the coast of Turkey, and more recently Croatia.

For the worker living in greater London, Venice today is almost as accessible as Brighton was 100 years ago. Consequently, the British seaside resort experienced a marked decline from the 1970s onwards. Some, such as New Brighton, Merseyside have disappeared. Others have reinvented themselves, and now cater to daytrippers and the weekend break market.

RECENT DEVELOPMENTS

There has been a discernible upmarket trend in tourism over the last few decades, especially in Europe where international travel for short breaks is commonplace. Tourists have higher levels of disposable income and greater leisure time. They are also better educated and have more sophisticated tastes. There is now a demand for a better quality product in many quarters. This has resulted in the following trends:-

- The old 'sun, sea, and sand' mass market has fragmented. People want more specialised versions of it, such as 'Club 18-30', quieter resorts with select hotels, self-catering, etc.
- People are taking second holidays in the form of short breaks/city breaks, ranging from British and European cities to country hotels.
- There has been a growth in niche markets catering for special interests or activities, including growth of destination hotels.

The developments in technology and transport infrastructure (particularly the advent of jumbo jets) have placed some types of holiday in the affordable mainstream:-

- The development of a mass cruise holiday market.
- The advent of affordable holidays to long-haul destinations such as Thailand or Kenya.
- The phenomenon of the low budget airline, utilising a new generation of small regional airports.

There have also been changes in lifestyle, which may call into question the current definitions of tourism. Some people (particularly the 45+ and retired) may be adopting a tourism lifestyle, living as a tourist all the year round-eating out several times a week, going to the theatre, daytripping, and indulging in short breaks several times a year.

Much of this results in impulse purchasing. This is facilitated by internet purchasing of tourism products. Some sites have now started to offer dynamic packaging, in which an inclusive price is quoted for a tailor-made package requested by the customer upon impulse.

There have been a few setbacks in tourism, such as the September 11, 2001 attacks and terrorist threats to tourist destinations such as Bali and European cities. Some of the tourist destinations, including the Costa del Sol, the Baleares and Cancún have lost popularity due to shifting tastes. In this context, the excessive building and environmental destruction often associated with traditional "sun and beach" tourism may contribute to a destination's saturation and subsequent decline. This appears to be the case with Spain's Costa Brava, a byword for this kind of tourism in the 1960s and 1970s. With only 11% of the Costa Brava now unblemished by low-quality development (Greenpeace Spain's figure), the destination now faces a crisis in its tourist industry. Sustainable tourism is becoming more popular as people start to realize the devastating effects tourism can have on communities.

Receptive tourism is now growing at a very rapid rate in many developing countries, where it is often the most important economic activity in local GDP. In recent years, second holidays or vacations have become more popular as people's discretionary income increases. Typical combinations are a package to the typical mass tourist resort, with a winter skiing holiday or weekend break to a city or national park.

On December 26, 2004 a tsunami, caused by the 2004 Indian Ocean earthquake hit Asian countries bordering the Indian Ocean, and also the Maldives. Tens of thousands of lives were lost, and many tourists died. This, together with the vast clean-up operation in place, has stopped or severely hampered tourism to the area.

SPECIAL FORMS OF TOURISM

For the past few decades other forms of tourism, also known as niche tourism, have been becoming more popular, particularly:

- Adventure tourism: tourism involving travel in rugged regions, or adventurous sports such as mountaineering and hiking (tramping).

- Agritourism: farm based tourism, helping to support the local agricultural economy.
- Ancestry tourism: (also known as genealogy tourism) is the travel with the aim of tracing one's ancestry, visiting the birth places of these ancestors and sometimes getting to know distant family.
- Armchair tourism and virtual tourism: not travelling physically, but exploring the world through internet, books, TV, etc.
- Audio tourism: includes audio walking tours and other audio guided forms of tourism including museum audio guides and audio travel books.
- Bookstore Tourism is a grassroots effort to support independent bookstores by promoting them as a travel destination.
- Creative Tourism is a new form of tourism that allows visitors to develop their creative potential, and get closer to local people, through informal participation in hands-on workshops that draw on the culture of their holiday destinations.
- Cultural tourism: includes urban tourism, visiting historical or interesting cities, and experiencing their cultural heritages. This type of tourism may also include specialized cultural experiences, such as art museum tourism where the tourist visits many art museums during the tour, or opera tourism where the tourist sees many operas or concerts during the tour.
- Coastal Tourism involves tourist products located along Coastal Environments-due to the limited extent of coastal environments they often are amongst the first places to experience coastal tourist congestion for a region.
- Dark tourism: is the travel to sites associated with death and suffering. The first tourist agency to specialise in this kind of tourism started with trips to Lakehurst, New Jersey, the scene of the Hindenburg airship disaster.

- Disaster tourism: travelling to a disaster scene not primarily for helping, but because it is interesting to see. It can be a problem if it hinders rescue, relief and repair work.
- Drug tourism: travel to a country to obtain or consume drugs, either legally or illegally.
- Ecotourism: sustainable tourism which has minimal impact on the environment, such as safaris (Kenya), Rainforests (Belize) and hiking (Lapland), or national parks.
- Educational tourism: may involve travelling to an education institution, a wooded retreat or some other destination in order to take personal-interest classes, such as cooking classes with a famous chef or crafts classes.
- Extreme tourism: tourism associated with high risk.
- Free Independent Traveler: a sector of the market and philosophy of constructing a vacation by sourcing one's own components eg accommodation, transport.
- Gambling tourism, e.g. to Atlantic City, Las Vegas, Palm Springs, California, Macau or Monte Carlo for the purpose of gambling at the casinos there.
- Garden tourism visiting botanical gardens famous places in the history of gardening, such as Versailles and the Taj Mahal.
- Heritage tourism: visiting historical (Rome, Athens, Cracow) or industrial sites, such as old canals, railways, battlegrounds, etc.
- Health tourism: usually to escape from cities or relieve stress, perhaps for some 'fun in the sun', etc. Often to Sanatoriums or "health spas".
- Hobby tourism: tourism alone or with groups to participate in hobby interests, to meet others with similar interests, or to experience something pertinent to the hobby. Examples might be garden tours, amateur radio DX-peditions, or square dance cruises.

- Inclusive tourism: tourism marketed to those with functional limits or disabilities. Referred to as "Tourism for All" in some regions. Destinations often employ Universal Design and Universal Destination Development principles.
- Mass Tourism is an ecotourism policy to minimise the footprint of tourists by concentrating them into a small area. Mass tourism also maximises the ultisation of tourist infrastructure.
- Medical tourism, e.g.:
  * for what is illegal in one's own country, such as abortion or euthanasia
  * for advanced care that is not available in one's own country
  * in the case that there are long waiting lists in one's own country
  * for use of free or cheap health care organisations
- Mystical tourism: Tourism for people that believe feel energy and travel to places to meditate, yoga, special events, ceremonies, mystical rituals.
- Pop-culture tourism: tourism by those that visit a particular location after reading about it or seeing it in a film.
- Perpetual tourism: individuals always on vacation; some of them, for tax purposes, to avoid being resident in any country.
- Pilgrimage Tourism: pilgrimages to ancient holy places (Rome and Santiago de Compostela for Catholics, temples and stupas of Nepal for the Hindus and Buddhist, Mount Athos or Painted churches of northern Moldavia for the Orthodox), religious sites such as mosques, shrines, etc.
- Sex tourism: travelling solely for the purpose of sexual activity, usually with prostitutes

- Shopping tourism promoting shopping festivals as tourist drawcards such as the Dubai, Singapore, Hong Kong and the Gold Coast.
- Solo Travel: travelling alone
- Sport travel: skiing, golf and scuba diving are popular ways to spend a vacation. This could also include travelling to a major international sporting event such as the FIFA World Cup or following a tour such as the Ashes or British and Irish Lions.
- Space tourism: traveling in outer space or on spaceships.
- Vacilando is a special kind of wanderer for whom the process of travelling is more important than the destination.
- Wine tourism, the visiting of growing regions, vineyards, wineries, tasting rooms, wine festivals, and similar places or events for the purpose of consuming or purchasing wine.

TRENDS

The World Tourism Organization (UNWTO) forecasts that international tourism will continue growing at the average annual rate of 4 %. By 2020 Europe will remain the most popular destination, but its share will drop from 60 % in 1995 to 46 %. Long-haul will grow slightly faster than intraregional travel and by 2020 its share will increase from 18 % in 1995 to 24 %.

With the advent of e-commerce, tourism products have become one of the most traded items on the internet. Tourism products and services have been made available through intermediaries, although tourism providers (hotels, airlines, etc.) can sell their services directly. This has put pressure on intermediaries from both on-line and traditional shops.

Space tourism is expected to "take off" in the first quarter of the 21st century, although compared with traditional destinations the number of tourists in orbit will remain low until technologies such as a space elevator make space travel cheap.

Technological improvement is likely to make possible air-ship hotels, based either on solar-powered airplanes or large dirigibles. Underwater hotels, such as Hydropolis, expected to open in Dubai in 2006, will be built. On the ocean tourists will be welcomed by ever larger cruise ships and perhaps floating cities.

Some futurists expect that movable hotel "pods" will be created that could be temporarily erected anywhere on the planet, where building a permanent resort would be unacceptable politically, economically or environmentally.

The term backpacking is said to have originated in the early 1970s with the advent of low-cost jet airplane fares. During this era it became common for young Westerners, to follow the hippie trail into India and Southeast Asia. This period also gave birth to the first budget guidebooks (see Tony and Maureen Wheeler) and began to change the way that many people looked at the possibilities and opportunities of travel.

More recently, backpacking has become something of a rite of passage in the popular culture of some countries, most notably Australia, Israel and New Zealand where after finishing high school, university or a period in the army they take several months to two year's break in Europe (some of whom work in this region), Asia or the Americas.

This can be put down to the light population and geographic isolation of these two countries from much of the world's population and history, the fact that Australia and New Zealand are both affluent English-speaking countries where the majority of their citizens can afford overseas travel, and that both countries have a tradition of students attending university in the home city rather than moving away for college.

A substantial amount of young adults from Israel also undertake long-term backpacking trips, particularly after they finish their mandatory military service. Travel of a backpacking nature is also extremely popular with Northern Europeans, particularly the Dutch and British and with small sections of North Americans and Japaneses.

CULTURE

Low-cost options are popular: such as sharing lifts, budget flights, rail/bus passes (or if the backpacking trip is circumglobal, a relatively cheap round-the-world air ticket which permits numerous stops), youth hostels, free hospitality services and buying food at local stores abroad instead of going to restaurants.

Hostels and other budget accommodations in the 'developed' world tend to be communal to some degree, and thus backpacker culture is often highly social and emphasizes the camaraderie of communal life, such as the shared kitchens common in many hostels. When backpackers stay in one place for a while, they often seek a house-share with numerous other backpackers and are likely to share a room to keep the costs down. In the 'developing' world accommodation is normally found in cheap hotels, pensions or guesthouses.

The common language of backpackers is overwhelmingly English in varying levels of fluency while German is arguably the second most common language encountered due to the large presence of backpackers from Germany or Switzerland. (However, German-speakers will usually only speak German informally amongst one another, and will otherwise speak English in most other situations). Britons, Australians, Canadians and Germans typically form among the most common backpacker nationalities in the world, in addition to Israelis, Americans, New Zealanders and numerous other Western European nations such as Switzerland or The Netherlands. Backpackers from Spain are very common in Latin America, where there is little or no language barriers and the cost of travel and living expenses is often very favorable for the Spanish. The same is true of French in West Africa. Per head of population, Australia is thought to have the highest representation of backpackers, although there is no data available to demonstrate this empirically.

Backpacker culture is perhaps typified by the Lonely Planet (Australian) series of guidebooks, which caters to budget travelers both in its regular guides as well as, more specifically, the "On a Shoestring" regional compilations. The Rough Guide (UK) and Let's Go (USA) series of guidebooks are also popular.

In France, the traditional backpacker's guidebook is the Guide du routard. Traditionally, backpackers do not travel with expensive electronic equipment such as laptop computers and PDAs due to concerns about theft, damage, and additional luggage weight. However, the desire to stay connected coupled with trends in lightweight electronics have given rise to the flashpacking trend. Some backpackers take a high resolution digital camera and/or high capacity MP3 Player with them on their travels. Blogging from various Internet cafes around the world is also a growing phenomenon, offering a more convenient way to relay information to interested friends and family at home.

AGE OF BACKPACKERS

Backpackers can be of any age to theoretically be part of the backpacker scene and subculture; however, the vast majority of budget travelers are clearly in their 20s. Patrons at most youth hostels are rarely under 18 (some even mandate a minimum age of 18) while guests over 30 constitute a minority. The 'stereotypical' backpacker is often envisioned as a senior college student or recent college graduate about 20 to 25 years of age with no dependents (spouse, children, etc.), therefore making it relatively easy to put typical daily responsibilities on temporary hiatus to go traveling for up to many months at a time. Depending on the part of the world people backpack through, the median age can vary slightly.

Philosophy

Rolf Potts writes in his book Vagabonding about what he sees as the myths that surround conventional travel: Of all the outrageous throwaway lines one hears in movies, there is one that stands out for me. It doesn't come from a madcap comedy, an esoteric science-fiction flick, or a special-effects-laden action thriller. It comes from Oliver Stone's Wall Street, when the Charlie Sheen character-a promising big shot in the stock market-is telling his girlfriend about his dreams.

> *"I think if I can make a bundle of cash before I'm thirty and get out of this racket," he says, "I'll be able to ride my motorcycle across China."*

When I first saw this scene on video a few years ago, I nearly fell out of my seat in astonishment. After all, Charlie Sheen or anyone else could work for eight months as a toilet cleaner and have enough money to ride a motorcycle across China. Even if they didn't yet have their own motorcycle, another couple months of scrubbing toilets would earn them enough to buy one when they got to China.

For many, this sums up the allure of backpacking, promising an "exotic" or "adventurous" experience that is also deemed "authentic," that is, an experience that, because it is self-planned and directed, does not fit within the typical Western-style vacation or travel industry.

This desire to experience "authentic" travel may be a reaction to the commercialization of the travel industry. Many backpackers express disdain towards "packaged" travel experiences including cruise ships and guided or bus tours which typically consist of a large number of tourists led by a guide. In contrast, backpacker philosophy encourages self-reliance and individuality, like overcoming the language barrier without the help of a translator or making all of one's own travel arrangements (to present two examples). John Gregory sums up this philosophy as:

Those spending big bucks for guided travel get peace-of-mind in return. They are guaranteed no worries, no hassles, an experience as close as possible to being home, without being home. They get an hour and fifteen minutes for the guaranteed-open museum, then a two-hour sightseeing ride that catches all the picture-postcard highlights.

They break for lunch at a "recommended" restaurant, where the food is reasonable and ordering is easy. And as the next bus pulls in they re-board theirs to repeat the routine, ending with an easy check-in at a reasonable hotel, populated with plenty of other tourists, pretty much like themselves.

While all travel is good for the human spirit, budget backpacking is unparalleled for meeting people and experiencing worlds on their own intimate terms. There are many travelers who have the resources for pampered-class but choose to strap on a backpack and see the world via the seat-of-their-pants, because they know it's the best way to experience cultures and interact with local people

In the United States among many other Western countries, this backlash against the large-scale commercial travel industry as expressed in the philosophy of backpacking has made some inroads into mainstream culture, such as in the popular travel guide writer Rick Steves who, like Tony and Maureen Wheeler of Lonely Planet, spun his experiences as a backpacker in the 1970s into a successful guidebook series.

In addition to notions of authenticity, some backpackers value the sense of freedom and independence in this mode of travel. Especially on extended trips, there is often only a rough itinerary, which can be changed at will. If a backpacker does not like a place, she can move on. If she likes it, she is free to stay and kick back for a while. Travel directions may change when a backpacker meets other independent travelers and learns about destinations she had not considered before or joins up with new friends. The semblance of "gypsy" life has its own romantic allure.

Of course, while backpack travel is carefree in this respect, it is more complicated in that backpackers have to plan everything and deal with all adversities themselves. There is no cruise director taking care of them. However, some backpackers also view this as a positive: It is a challenge and adventure, and the sometimes intense problem-solving in unfamiliar surroundings helps to hone their life skills.

WORKING ON THE ROAD

Many backpackers gain temporary work (usually low-paid, unskilled, casual, and sometimes in violation of local labor laws) in the countries they visit. For instance, London's pubs are well known for the number of Australian bartenders working in them; "Irish pubs" around the world hire Irish backpackers. In Australia, fruit picking is a popular job among backpackers, although it can be physically demanding. Although while staying in one place for a long duration, say while working and living in semi-permanent accommodation it could be questioned whether you are still backpacking in the form of the adjective. Backpackers are also commonly employed by hostels, where English-language proficiency and familiarity with hostel operations are considered assets. Hostels around the world are increasing their revenue by inaugurating work and travel programs, where hostelers can work for accommodation by performing basic hostel upkeep and operational duties.

CRITICISM

Backpacker philosophy is sometimes criticized for being hypocritical. Some travelers have been known to forego finding "authentic" contact with a culture, and instead congregate only with other travelers in international hostels or guesthouses.

In addition, backpackers are sometimes blamed for the commercialization of the destinations they travel to. By definition, any "undiscovered paradise" cannot remain pristine under the demand of thousands of visitors. This can often lead to the overuse of certain natural and cultural resources, a vice backpacking shares with other forms of tourism. A notable example of this phenomenon is Byron Bay in Australia, which was a largely quiet backpacker town in the 1970s and is now considered one of the most popular destinations in the 2000s with a bias for yuppies. This is sometimes said to actually pervert the backpacking culture itself: while backpackers seek genuineness and "authentic" cultural interactions, thus often looking for places with as few other foreigners as possible, they very often tend to meet in so-called "backpacker paradises"- places where all backpackers meet and that, eventually, end-up being modern-day "hippie-resorts". Examples include San Pedro de Atacama, a formerly isolated village in Chile and now a town dependent on tourism. This phenomenon is perhaps not unlike the phenomenon of gentrification that happens in urban ecologies.

A third layer of criticism is economic. Backpackers' pursuit of "cheap" travel destinations is only possible through the imbalance of living costs between Western and developing nations. Thus, backpacking can be seen as an inherently exploitative activity that benefits from the poverty of destination countries. Bolivia and Cambodia are notable examples of very inexpensive countries which backpackers visit and have the ability to stay comfortably for months even on a relatively small budget, all the while contributing little to the local have-nots. A more recent example includes the collapse of the peso currency in Argentina in the early 2000s, which quickly made that country a very attractive destination for budget backpackers. However, backpackers, involved as they are in an inherently pragmatic project, rarely give this concern any more thought than it deserves.

The idea that the passing of money from the more affluent to the less affluent is "exploitative" is not as compelling as it may have been in decades past. A more plausible economic criticism, from the point of view of the local economy, is that backpackers do not spend as much money as packaged or luxury tourists.

ADVANTAGES

In their defense, some backpackers say that budget travel pumps money into the economies of Third World countries, increasing their standard of living and creating jobs, and doing this in a way that is inherently more egalitarian than mainstream tour companies, who often operate with minimal contact with third party vendors or average citizens. Backpacking in comparison, frequently makes use of local food vendors, merchants and accommodations, and thus does more to benefit the local economy. The lower cost to the budget-conscious young Western tourist and the increased patronage to local merchants actually makes the economics of backpacking a win-win situation in many cases.

Backpackers are accused of traveling to exotic places only to associate with other backpackers. That perception is probably correct but requires some explanation. Generally backpackers are from developed countries, speak fluent English (even if from a non-English speaking country). When these backpackers arrive in developing countries they congregate at the hostels and guesthouses in the center of town where they tend to not blend in. In these areas the best English speakers among the locals tend to be touts who will prey upon the backpackers to visit the factories that they "own", to buy jewels to smuggle back and resell in their home countries, to purchase their services as a "guide" and to undertake illegal activities such as gambling, prostitution and drug use.

Most backpackers would like to interact with locals, but have a hard time fending off the touts, as bargaining and negotiating hassle are key factors of backpacking in parts of the world. Locals with the intent of approaching a backpacker are generally not as aggressive as the touts. Backpackers would consider it obtrusive to approach a local in English and ask to join the local in their home for dinner for instance. The inability to travel beyond the areas covered by public transportation further strain the situation.

'DEVELOPED' AND 'DEVELOPING' WORLD DESTINATIONS

It is worth noting that there is a notable difference between backpacking travel in the developed world, typically Australia, New Zealand, North America and Europe where hostel are commonly used, than in the developing world, typically South and South-East Asia, Africa and Latin America. In such developing nations travel is cheaper, but often harder. Equally where backpacking is popular, whole industries have established to tend to the needs of backpackers offering services to make their lives easier (laundry, visa applications, train tickets) and goods from 'home' countries not commonly available such as Falafel for Israelis, Marmite/vegemite for British/Australian. Plus bars/restaurants showing sporting events from 'back home' and bootleg copies of movies. Well know examples of such places would be the Khaosan Road in Bangkok, Anjuna in Goa and Antigua in Guatemala. In backpacker hot-spots, many bars and restaurants are set up primary for backpackers with few locals patronizing them-this again fosters the social aspect of backpacking travel.

Favourite

Classically, Western Europe is a very common backpacker destination because of the availability of public transport and the large number of hostels and other budget accommodations. However, since the fall of the Berlin Wall and the dissolution of the Soviet states, Eastern Europe has become a rapidly growing destination for budget travelers. Originally this meant cities such as Prague and Budapest, but more recently Croatia, Slovenia, the Balkans, and the Baltic Republics have become a popular stops on the backpacking circuit

Long-term backpacker destinations are places in the developing world with low costs of living such as Goa (India), Essaouira (Morocco), or Thailand. Australia's East Coast is also a very popular destination for many backpackers. Latin America is quickly becoming a hot-spot for backpackers, who are drawn to the continent by the often favorable exchange rates and unique culture and beauty. Machu Picchu, Patagonia, the Triple Frontier and the cities of Buenos Aires, Rio de Janeiro, La Paz and Cusco are often the highlights for travelers to this continent and see the most 'traffic'.

As mentioned above, certain destinations are so popular on the backpacking circuit that some cities house "backpacker ghettos," whole districts where large numbers of travellers congregate to find cheap accommodation, street food, and share travel information. The most famous of these is the Khaosan Road area of downtown Bangkok.

It is true to say that most backpacking follows established routes with terms such as the 'gringo trail' in Latin America and the 'Banana Pancake' or trail' in Southeast Asia used. These routes and popular countries generally focus on three factors. One reputation, what is the current hot destination? Two popular sights that everyone seems to want to see: Machu Picchu, the Sydney Opera House, Prague, etc. And finally round the world air travel routing and airline hubs.

It is easy to argue that Thailand's huge popularity is in no small measure a result of (it's ease of travel and natural beauty aside) the fact it is an obvious stop-off between Europe and Australia. Consider the Philippines which has no overland connections, is not a major stop-off and holds similar attributes to Thailand is far less popular. The same is true of Eastern Europe's and Central America's proximity to affluent Western

Europe and North America. Africa and notably, West Africa see relativity few backpackers since including them in a round-the-world ticket is difficult and expensive.

Avoided

While largely a matter of nationality, personal taste and the current political situation, some generalizations can be made about the destinations many backpackers avoid. For example, a fair number of backpackers, like many other tourists, avoid countries where there is a perceived danger of terrorism, food poisoning or hassle in the way of getting a visa or repeatedly being accosted to purchase goods/services. Some countries, wising up to what's good for their travel economy, have tried to address these issues. Morocco, which at some point had one of the worst reputations in this regard, is reported to have clamped down on hustling and touting aimed at foreign travelers. In Asia and Eastern Europe visa regulations are being greatly relaxed encourage more travelers. In Egypt, Turkey and Pakistan huge efforts are made to safe-guard travelers from terrorism and countries such as Syria and Iran, while holding terrible reputations abroad are welcoming of backpackers (once issued with a visa).

High Costs

Regions with a high cost of living, such as Scandinavia for example, are avoided by many long-term backpackers because of the expense. Other destinations have high costs for transportation, such as Polynesia, and are also avoided by the majority of backpackers. This rule applies to a lesser degree to many destinations in Western Europe, where costs are generally high enough to discourage extensive (three months and longer) budget travel. Travel to popular but extremely expensive cities such as New York City or London is generally limited to just several days, and backpackers tend to try and fit as much daily sight-seeing as possible in such locations.

Infrastructure

While not an absolute, countries without developed infrastructure, especially in the form of public transportation, are more difficult for backpackers to travel in because of the serious limits on mobility. This includes many African countries and the greater part of Central Asia. Some travellers also avoid the United States of America for similar reasons, because of the general lack of public transport, the expense of renting a car and the lack of hostels in many destinations, which are largely relegated only to the most major cities, the California Coast, parts of New England, and parts of Florida. Hostels in the United States are also generally expensive in comparison to many other countries, often between $US20-30 per night.

This has given the United States a reputation for being relatively 'unfriendly' towards backpacking culture even though it is a highly desirable, varied, and generally safe country to be explored for foreign backpackers. The prevalence of motel chains, catering primarily to private motorists, may contribute to the relatively small number of backpacker hostels in the USA. These same problems are also present to an extent in parts of Canada, where the centrally-located provinces generally have few options for backpackers. People who wish to travel the United States extensively and as cheaply as possible often decide to purchase an economical van with improvised bedding within the vehicle. Even this option is becoming increasingly expensive however, as oil prices in the 2000s remain stubbornly high. This lifestyle also may discourage many solo backpackers, as they must pay many bills entirely by themselves and establish few social connections.

Instability

While the desire to travel at low cost and the desire to travel with convenience and security are often at odds, some countries are generally avoided by backpackers because of the general political instability. In the most extreme cases, such as Iraq, Somalia or North Korea opportunities for travel may be severely curtailed or an outright impossibility. Other areas are avoided by many backpackers because of the perceived general hostility of the political climate, including some parts of the Middle East and Central Asia, Myanmar and parts of Central Africa.

These are generalizations made by the majority of the community and are disputed by many others (Myanmar being a recent example of debate), especially travelers drawn to "dangerous" destinations.

Crime, Dangers and Victimization

Some countries are largely avoided by backpackers due to a substantially increased risk of being kidnapped or mugged of their possessions, to the point where the benefits of travel may not compensate for their dangers. Colombia in South America is a notable example, which has the unfortunate reputation of having one of the highest number of kidnappings per capita in the world. Many other South American cities, such as Rio de Janeiro, São Paulo and Lima, also have high crime rates. Moreover, African cities such as Johannesburg or Nairobi are also discouraged on the backpacker circuit due to their high crime rates and perceived danger of visiting.

Generally a backpacker will keep his main funds and important documents in the hostel or guesthouse room or safe to minimize damage if robbed or lost during the day. Backpackers are thus most vulnerable when traveling between locations when they are carrying all their belongings and items most often go missing on public transport or at bus/train stations.

Traveling by day will always minimize this risk as does being careful and/or in a group. It seems backpackers universally trust other backpackers based on the logic that someone wouldn't come all the way from [Stockholm, Berlin, Sydney, etc.] just to steal from other tourists (Although the wisdom of this logic is drawn into question due to the desperate financial woes often encountered by poorly planned backpackers). On the whole dangers while backpacking, when put in perspective and if using common sense are not overly great (certainly lower than that of the dangers of road traffic accidents, in many parts of the world), but unfortunately some travelers are either over confident, don't exercise common sense or (the minority) unlucky and fall victim to some annoyance.

Health is another issue of concern for backpackers with sometimes poor health facilities away from urban hubs and prevalence of diseases such as in some regions, malaria. More common, however are minor ailments like sun burn, diarrhea or food poisoning, which seems to be an unfortunate caveat of third world travel.

Crowds

Many backpackers try to avoid crowds of other (ordinary) tourists. The first rule is to avoid traditional package holiday destinations such as Benidorm or Cancún because it goes against the backpacker's image. Such places may also be undesirable because of high costs, inauthentic culture, limited sightseeing options and exclusively prebooked accommodation.

Language Barriers

While a matter of personal taste, willingness to learn foreign languages, and other stipulations, countries where the English language is not widely understood or holds little sway in everyday life can or cannot be seen as a hinderence for independent travel. This may include a significant part of Latin America, many parts of Africa, Central Asia, and more rural areas of East Asia. However, this can also be seen as challenging, so it can just as well draw many backpackers to these regions.

HOTEL

The 4-star Manor House Hotel at Castle Combe, Wiltshire, England. Built in the fourteenth century, the hotel has 48 rooms and 365 acres (1.5 km^2) of gardens. The Las Vegas Strip is lined with the world's largest hotels, most of which have a 4-or 5-star rating and over 2,000 rooms each. A hotel is an establishment that provides paid lodging, usually on a short-term basis. Hotels often provide a number of additional guest services such as a restaurant, a swimming pool or childcare. Some hotels have conference services and meeting rooms and encourage groups to hold conventions and meetings at their location.

Hotels differ from motels in that most motels have drive-up, exterior entrances to the rooms, while hotels tend to have interior entrances to the rooms, which may increase guests' safety and present a more upmarket image.

In Australia, a hotel may also be an establishment that serves alcoholic drinks, and usually meals in a casual setting but which does not necessarily provide accommodation. This type of establishment would more usually be called a pub or bar in other countries. In general use in Australia the terms '"hotel" and pub are usually taken to be synonymous. In India, the word may also refer to a restaurant since the best restaurants were always situated next to a good hotel.

Origins of the Term

The word hotel derives from the French hôtel, which referred to a French version of a townhouse, not a place offering accommodation (in contemporary usage, hôtel has the meaning of "hotel", and hôtel particulier is used for the old meaning). The French spelling (with the circumflex) was once also used in English, but is now rare. The circumflex replaces the 's' once preceding the 't' in the earlier hostel spelling, which over time received a new, but closely related meaning.

Services and Facilities

Basic accommodation of a room with only a bed, a cupboard, a small table and a washstand has largely been replaced by rooms with en-suite bathrooms and, more commonly in the United States than elsewhere, climate control. Other features found may be a telephone, an alarm clock, a TV, and broadband Internet connectivity. Food and drink may be supplied by a mini-bar (which often includes a small refrigerator) containing snacks and drinks (to be paid for on departure), and tea and coffee making facilities (cups, spoons, an electric kettle and sachets containing instant coffee, tea bags, sugar, and creamer or milk). In the United Kingdom a hotel is required by law to serve food and drinks to all comers within certain stated hours; to avoid this requirement it is not uncommon to come across "private hotels" which are not subject to this requirement. However, in Japan the capsule hotel supplies minimal facilities and room space.

Classification

The cost and quality of hotels are usually indicative of the range and type of services available. Due to the enormous increase in tourism worldwide during the last decades of the 20th century, standards, especially those of smaller establishments, have improved considerably. For the sake of greater comparability, rating systems have been introduced, with the one to five stars classification being most common.

Boutique Hotels

"Boutique Hotel" is a term originating in North America to describe intimate, usually luxurious or quirky hotel environments. Boutique hotels differentiate themselves from larger chain or branded hotels by providing an exceptional and personalized level of accommodation, services and facilities.

Boutique hotels are furnished in a themed, stylish and/or aspirational manner. Although usually considerably smaller than a mainstream hotel (ranging from 3 to 100 guest rooms) boutique hotels are generally fitted with telephone and wi-fi Internet connections, honesty bars and often cable/pay TV. Guest services are attended to by 24 hour hotel staff. Many boutique hotels have on site dining facilities, and the majority offer bars and lounges which may also be open to the general public. Of the total travel market a small percentage are discerning travelers, who place a high importance on privacy, luxury and service delivery. As this market is typically corporate travelers, the market segment is non-seasonal, high-yielding and repeat, and therefore one which boutique hotel operators target as their primary source of income.

Famous Hotels

Some hotels have gained their renown through tradition, by hosting significant events or persons, such as Schloss Cecilienhof in Potsdam, Germany, which derives its fame from the so-called Potsdam Conference of the World War II allies Winston Churchill, Harry Truman and Joseph Stalin in 1945. Other establishments have given name to a particular meal or beverage, as is the case with the Waldorf Astoria in New York City, USA, known for its Waldorf Salad or the Raffles Hotel in Singapore, where the drink Singapore Sling was invented. Another example is the Hotel Sacher in Vienna Austria, home of the Sachertorte. There are also hotels which became much more popular through films like the Grand Hotel Europe in Saint Petersburg, Russia when James Bond stayed there in the Blockbuster, Goldeneye. Cannes hotels such as the Carlton or the Martinez become the center of the world during Cannes Film Festival (France).

A number of hotels have entered the public consciousness through popular culture, such as the Ritz Hotel in London, UK ('Putting on The Ritz') and Hotel Chelsea in New York City, subject of a number of songs and also the scene of the alleged stabbing of Nancy Spungen by her boyfriend Sid Vicious. Hotels that enter folklore like these two are also often frequented by celebrities, as is the case both with the Ritz and the Chelsea. Other famous hotels include the Beverly Hills Hotel, the Hotel Bel-Air and the Chateau Marmont, in California, Watergate complex in Washington DC, the Hotel Astoria in Saint Petersburg, Russia, the Hotel George V and Hôtel Ritz in Paris, Palazzo Versace hotel on the Gold Coast, Queensland, Australia, Hotel Hermitage and Hotel de Paris in Monaco (in the French Riviera), Peninsula Hotel in Hong Kong and Hotel Leningradskaya in Moscow.

Unusual Hotels

Many hotels can be considered destinations in themselves, by dint of unusual features of the lodging and/or its immediate environment:

Treehouse Hotels

Some hotels, such as the Costa Rica Tree House in the Gandoca-Manzanillo Wildlife Refuge, Costa Rica, or Treetops Hotel in Aberdare National Park, Kenya, are built with living trees as structural elements, making them treehouses. The Ariau Towers near Manaus, Brazil is in the middle of the Amazon, on the Rio Negro. Bill Gates even invested and had a suite built there with satellite internet/phone. Another hotel with treehouse units is Bayram's Tree Houses in Olympos, Turkey.

Cave Hotels

Desert Cave Hotel in Coober Pedy, South Australia and the Cuevas Pedro Antonio de Alarcón (named after the author) in

Guadix, Spain, as well as several hotels in Cappadocia, Turkey, are notable for being built into natural cave formations, some with rooms underground.

Capsule Hotels

Capsule hotels are a type of economical hotels that are quite common in Japan.

Ice Hotels

Ice hotels, such as the Ice Hotel in Jukkasjärvi, Sweden, melt every spring and are rebuilt out of ice and snow each winter.

Snow Hotels

The Mammut Snow Hotel in Finland is located within the walls of the Kemi snow castle, which is the biggest in the world. It includes The Mammut Snow Hotel, The Castle Courtyard, The Snow Restaurant and a chapel for weddings, etc. Its furnishings and its decorations, such as sculptures, are made of snow and ice. There is snow accommodation also in Lainio Snow Hotel in Lapland (near Ylläs), Finland.

Garden Hotels

Garden hotels, famous for their gardens before they became hotels, includes Gravetye Manor, the home of William Robinson and Cliveden, designed by Charles Barry with a rose garden by Geoffrey Jellicoe.

Underwater Hotels

As of 2005, the only hotel with an underwater room that can be reached without Scuba diving is Utter Inn in Lake Mälaren, Sweden. It only has one room, however, and Jules' Undersea Lodge in Key Largo, Florida, which requires scuba diving, is not much bigger.

Hydropolis is an ambitious project to build a luxury hotel in Dubai, UAE, with 220 suites, all on the bottom of the Persian Gulf, 20 meters (66 feet) below the surface. Its architecture will feature two domes that break the surface and an underwater train tunnel, all made of transparent materials such as glass and acrylic.

Other unusual Hotels

The Library Hotel in New York City is unique in that its ten floors are arranged according to the Dewey Decimal System.

The Rogers Centre, formerly SkyDome, in Toronto, Canada is the only stadium to have a hotel connected to it, with 70 rooms overlooking the field.

The Burj al-Arab hotel in Dubai, United Arab Emirates, built on an artificial island, is structured in the shape of a sail of a boat. The RMS Queen Mary in Long Beach, California is the only 1930s ocean liner still in existence. Its elegant first-class staterooms are now used as a hotel. The Oriental Pearl Tower in Shanghai houses an extremely expensive hotel with only 20 rooms.

World-record Setting Hotels

Tallest

The tallest hotel in the world is the Burj al-Arab in Dubai, United Arab Emirates, at 321 metres, which however will soon be surpassed by the nearby Rose Rotana Suites at 333 meters (1,091 feet). The Ryugyong Hotel in Pyongyang was intended to reach 330 meters (1,083 feet), but is unlikely to be completed; it has been under construction since 1987 and was abandoned in 1992. The highest hotel rooms are in the Grand Hyatt in the Jin Mao Building in Shanghai, the highest floor being at around 350 m.

Largest

The largest hotel in the world is the MGM Grand Las Vegas in Las Vegas, Nevada, USA with a total of 6,276 rooms as of December 20, 2006. On December 18, 2006 Guinness World Records listed the First World Hotel in Genting Highlands, Malaysia as the worlds largest hotel. It has a total of 6,118 rooms and is part of the Genting Highlands Resort and Casino. The First World Plaza which is joined to the two hotel towers boasts 500,000 square feet of indoor theme park, shopping centres, casino gaming areas, and eateries. Previously, Guinness had listed the MGM Grand Las Vegas in Las Vegas, Nevada, USA with 5,005 rooms as the largest hotel in the world.

Oldest

According to the Guinness Book of World Records, the oldest hotel still in operation is the Hoshi Ryokan, in Awazu, Japan. It opened in 717, and features hot springs.

Hotel Occupations

The owner, chairman, or CEO of a hotel or hotel group is known as a hotelier.

Living in Hotels

The American billionaire Howard Hughes lived much of his life in hotels. He moved with his entourage from hotel to hotel and from Beverly Hills to Boston before deciding to move to Las Vegas and become a casino baron. Less than a month after his November 27, 1966 arrival, Hughes made a public offer to buy the Desert Inn.

The hotel's 8th floor became the nerve center of his empire and the 9th floor penthouse became Hughes's personal residence. Hughes moved to the Bahamas, Vancouver, London and several other locations-always taking up residence in the top floor penthouse of the hotel. Between 1966 and 1968, he also purchased several other hotel-casinos from the Mafia: Castaways, New Frontier, The Landmark Hotel and Casino, Sands and Silver Slipper.

Coco Chanel made the Hôtel Ritz in Paris her home for more than thirty years, until the day of her death, at 87, in a suite now named "Coco Chanel Suite". King Peter II of Yugoslavia spent much of the Second World War at Claridge's, a hotel in London. His son, Aleksandar Karadordevic, was born in the hotel. Prince Felix Yusupov lived in the Hotel Vendôme in Paris.

Alois Brunner, Austrian Nazi war criminal, is believed to have lived in the Meridian Hotel in Damascus, Syria, under the name Georg Fischer. Sultan Said Bin Taimur of Muscat lived at Dorchester Hotel in London after he was deposed by Qaboos of Oman in 1970, He died in the hotel in 1972. Eleftherios Venizelos, Greek statesman and diplomat, lived in the Hôtel Ritz Paris while he was in exile in France from 1935-1936.

Hotels in Fiction

Hotels have been chosen by authors as settings for crime fiction, farce and mystery works. A hotel is perfect as a mysterious, anonymous setting where various characters may gather. Hotels also feature in films, television series, songs and even theme park rides.

RESORT

A resort is a place used for relaxation or recreation, attracting visitors for holidays or vacations. Resorts are places, towns such as Newport, Rhode Island or St. Moritz, Switzerland, or larger regions, like the Adirondack Mountains or the Jersey Shore. A resort is not merely a commercial establishment operated by a single company, although in the late twentieth century this sort of faciltiy became more common. Such a self-contained resort attempts to provide for all or most of a vacationer's wants while remaining on the premises, such as food, drink, lodging, sports, entertainment, and shopping. The term "resort" sometimes is misused to identify a hotel that does not provide the other amenities required of a full resort. However, a hotel is frequently a central feature of a resort, such as the Grand Hotel at Mackinac Island, Michigan. Towns that contain resorts-or where tourism or vacationing is a major part of the local activity-are often called resort towns. The Walt Disney World Resort is a prominent example of a modern, self-contained commercial resort. Resorts exist throughout the world, increasingly attracting visitors from around the globe. Thailand, for instance, has become a popular destination. Resorts are especially prevalent in Central America and the Caribbean. Closely related to resorts are convention and large meeting sites. Generally these occur in cities where special meeting halls, together with ample accommodations as well as varied dining and entertainment are provided.

TYPES OF RESORTS

Resort at a Destination

A commercial establishment at a resort destinaton such as a recreational area, a scenic or historic site, a theme park, a gaming facility or other tourist attraction competes with other businesses at that destination.. Examples would be hotels in and around Disney World, resorts in St. Martin in the Caribbean, and establishments at Aspen, Colorado in the USA.

Destination Resort

A destination resort is a resort that contains, in and of itself, the necessary guest attraction capabilities-that is to say that a destination resort does not need to be near a destination (town, historic site, theme park, or other) to attract its public. Consequently, another characteristic of a destination resort is that is offers food, drink, lodging, sports, entertainment, and shopping within the facility so that guests have no need to leave the facility throughout their stay. Commonly these facilities are of higher quality than would be expected if one were to stay at a hotel or eat in a town's restaurants. Some examples are Atlantis in the Bahamas, Costa do Sauípe in the Northeastern Brazil, Laguna Phuket in Thailand and Sun City near Johannesburg in South Africa.

All-inclusive Resort

An all-inclusive resort is a resort that, besides providing all of the common amenities of a resort, charges a fixed price that includes most or all items. At a minimum, most inclusive resorts include lodging, unlimited food, drink, sports activities, and entertainment for the fixed price.

Historical Resorts

A famous resort of the ancient world was Baiae, Italy, popular over 2,000 years ago. Capri, an island near Naples, Italy, has attracted visitors since Roman times.

Medical tourism or medical travel, is the act of traveling to other countries to obtain medical, dental, and surgical care. The term was initially coined by travel agencies and the media as a catchall phrase to describe a rapidly growing industry where people travel to other countries to obtain medical care. Leisure aspect of traveling may be included on such a medical travel trip. It includes medical services (inclusive of elective procedure and complex specialised surgeries) like knee/hip replacement, heart surgery, dental procedures and different cosmetic surgeries. Many companies like Medical Excursions, Inc. inspect the overseas facilities and then help the North Amercian patients to find qualified affordable and high class medical service providers.

DESCRIPTION

A combination of many factors has led to the recent increase in popularity of medical travel: the high cost of healthcare in industrialized nations, the ease and affordability of international travel, and the improvement of technology and standards of care in many countries of the world. A large draw to medical travel is the convenience in comparison to that of other countries. Some countries that operate from a public health-care system are so taxed that it can take a considerable amount of time, to get needed medical care.

The time spent waiting for a procedure, such as a hip replacement, can be a year or more in Britain and Canada; however, in Singapore, Bangkok or Bangalore, a patient could feasibly have an operation the day after their arrival. Reasons pushing medical travel include lower healthcare costs as well as the search for medical expertise and safety. According to research found in an article by the University of Delaware publication, UDaily:

> *"the cost of surgery in Bolivia, Argentina, India, Thailand or South Africa can be one-tenth of what it is in the United States or Western Europe, and sometimes even less. A heart-valve replacement that would cost US$200,000 or more in the U.S., for example, goes for $10,000 in India-and that includes round-trip airfare and a brief vacation package. Similarly, a metal-free dental bridge worth $5,500 in the U.S. costs $500 in India or Bolivia, a knee replacement in Thailand with six days of physical therapy costs about one-fifth of what it would in the States, and Lasik eye surgery worth $3,700 in the U.S. is available in many other countries for only*

$730. Cosmetic surgery savings are even greater: A full facelift that would cost $20,000 in the U.S. runs about $2,500 in South Africa or $ 2,300 in bolivia."

To understand the phenomenon of Medical travel, we can compare the average costs of cosmetic surgeries between the industrialized nations and the most popular countries in latin america which are specialized in medical tourism and cosmetic surgery tourism (Argentina, Bolivia, Brazil, Costa Rica, India, Mexico). All the prices have been provided us by the offices affiliated with the ministries of health in USA, Europe (France, Spain, Switzerland), Argentine, Bolivia, brazil, Costa Rica, India, and Mexico. Medical tourists can come from anywhere in the world and may seek essential healthcare services such as cancer treatment and brain and transplant surgery as well as complementary or 'elective' services such as aesthetic treatments (cosmetic surgery). Popular Medical travel worldwilde destinations are: Singapore, India, Thailand, Brunei, Cuba, Hong Kong, Hungary, India, Israel, Jordan, Lithuania, Malaysia, The Philippines, Thailand, Singapore, and recently, UAE. Popular Cosmetic Surgery travel destination are:Argentina, Bolivia, Brazil, Costa Rica, Mexico and Turkey.

In Europe Belgium and Poland are also breaking into the business. South Africa is taking the term "medical tourism" very literally by promoting their "medical safaris": Come to see African wildlife and get a facelift in the same trip. However, feelings towards medical tourism are not always positive. In places like the US, where most have insurance and access to quality health care, medical tourism is viewed as risky. In some parts of the world, wider political issues can influence where medical tourists will choose to seek out healthcare; for example, in late 2006 some patients from the Middle East were choosing to travel to Singapore or Hong Kong for health care rather than to the USA.

While the tourism component might be a big draw for some Southeast Asia countries that focus on simple procedures, India is positioning itself the primary medical destination for the most complex medical procedures in the world. India's commitment to this is demonstrated with an ever growing number of hospitals that are attaining the US Joint Commission International accreditation. Singapore positions itself as a medical hub where healthcare services, medicine, biomedical research and pharmaceutical manufacturing converge. Singapore has made international news for many complex surgeries in specialties such as neurology, oncology and organ transplants procedures. Currently Singapore boasts the largest number of US Joint Commission accredited hospitals in the region. On the other hand, in South America, countries such as Argentina, Bolivia, Brazil lead on plastic surgery medical skills relying on the vast experience their surgeons have in treating the style-obsessed. It is estimated that 1 in 30 Argentinians had taken plastic surgery procedures, making this population the most operated in the world after the US and Mexico.

In Bolivia the situation is impressive. According to the "Sociedad Boliviana de Cirugia Plastica y Reconstructiva", more that 70% women who belong to the middle and upper class had taken plastic surgery procedure. There are companies emerging to offer global healthcare options that will allow North American patients to take full advantage of dramatic reductions in air travel and access world class healthcare at a fraction of the cost. Companies that focus on 'Medical Value Travel' typically will have experienced nurse case managers to assist patients with pre-and post-travel medical issues. They will also help provide resources for follow-up care upon the patient's return. While these services will initially be of interest to the self-insured patient, several studies indicate that the rapid growth of Health Savings Accounts will also drive interest to healthcare in other countries.

Because standards are everything when it comes to healthcare, there is a parallel issue around hospital accreditation. Potential medical tourists may be assisted in making their choices by whether or not hospitals have been assessed and accredited by reputable external accreditation bodies. In the USA, JCI (Joint Commission International) fulfills such a role, while in the United Kingdom and Hong Kong, the Trent Accreditation Scheme is a key player.

INDIA

India is one of the most touted destinations in the world for medical tourists. It is known in particular for heart surgery and hip resurfacing, areas of advanced medicine in which India is generally considered a global leader. Probably no country has been in the news for medical tourism than India in 2005-06, and the government and private hospital groups both seem committed to a goal of making the subcontinent a world leader in the industry. Indian medical industry's main appeal is low-cost treatment. Most estimates claim treatment costs in India start at around a tenth of the price of comparable treatment in America or Britain. Morever Indian Hospitals also provides more personalized care than available in west. For example, in April Madras Medical Mission, a Chennai-based hospital, successfully conducted a complex heart operation on an 87-year-old American patient at a reported cost of $8,000 (□7,000, £4,850) including the cost of his airfare and a month's stay in hospital.

The patient claimed that a less complex operation in America had earlier cost him $40,000. Take the rising popularity of "preventive health screening". At one private clinic in London a thorough men's health check-up that includes blood tests, electro-cardiogram tests, chest x-rays, lung tests and abdominal ultrasound costs £345 ($574, □500). By comparison, a comparable check-up at a clinic operated by Delhi-based healthcare company Max Healthcare costs $84. A lady from Vero beach, FL, who was featured in CBS 60 min in April 2005, went to India for hip surgery. In USA only hip replacements are possible, but India allows hip resurfacing that does not need the full hip replacement rather saves part of the hip to achieve the same result as the hip replacement.--Shyamvaran 00:57, 16 January 2007 (UTC)

Escorts Heart Institute and Research Center in Delhi and Faridabad, India performs nearly 15,000 heart operations every year, and the post-surgery mortality rate is only 0.8 percent, which is less than half of most major hospitals in the United States. Medical Tourism in India is one of the best options available to people across the globe. Millions come to India every year to get treated and then enjoy their recuperative holidays across India. People from different walks of life cut across America, United Kingdom, Pakistan, Sri Lanka, Europe, Maldives, Germany and numerous other countries come to India to have their treatments done with peace of mind.

India provides world class medical facilities with hospitals and specialized multi specialty health centers providing their expertise in the areas of Cosmetic Surgery, Dental care, Heart Surgeries, Coronary Bypass, Heart Check up, Valve replacements, Knee Replacements, Eye surgeries, Indian traditional treatments like Ayurvedic Therapies and much more, practically covering every aspect of medicine combining modern treatments with traditional experience. Estimates of the value of medical tourism to India go as high as $2 billion a year by 2012. In 2003, Indian finance minister Jaswant Singh called for India to become a "global health destination". However, the biggest stumbling block preventing the rapid growth of India as a healthcare destination is its poor infrastructure and lack of quality hotels.

SINGAPORE

Singapore's healthcare services built on a heritage of excellent quality, safety and trustworthiness, coupled with advanced research and international accreditation, and is Asia's leading medical hub. Nine hospitals and two medical centres in Singapore have obtained Joint Commission International (JCI) accreditation. JCI is the main hospital accreditation agency in the United States.

According to statistics at the official website, www.singaporemedicine.com, 374, 000 visitors came to Singapore purely to seek healthcare in 2005. Many of these patients come from neighbouring countries such as Indonesia and Malaysia. However, patient numbers from Indo-China, South-Asia, the Middle East and Greater China to Singapore are seeing fast growth. On top of that, patients from developed countries such as United States also choose Singapore as their medical travel destination for relatively affordable quality healthcare services in a clean cosmopolitan city for a peace of mind. Singapore made news for many complex and innovative procedures such as the separation of conjoined twins and tooth-in-eye surgery. The successful separation of the 10-month-old nepalese conjoined twins in 2001 puts Singapore's medical expertise onto the World's headlines. Singapore has since accomplished many more milestones both in Asia and in the world arena.

Recently, Singapore also hosted the first International Medical Travel Conference (IMTC) from 12th-15th December 2006. The four-day event attracted participants and media from 21 countries, setting pace and platform for the development of the budding medical travel industry. The conference aims to bring together thought leaders to examine some of the fundamentals, issues and challenges involved in the burgeoning international medical travel industry. Curiously however major media did not pay attention to this awkwardly managed event. However, up to late 2006 Singapore Hospitals have only chosen to accredit themselves through Joint Commission International (JCI), a US-based group, and this approach may have little appeal to potential health tourists based in other parts of the world. In time, Singapore Hospitals may look towards other European or Asian-based systems of hospital accreditation in an attempt to broaden their credibility and appeal.

THAILAND

Medical tourism is a growing segment of Thailand's tourism and health-care sectors. Lower labor costs translate into significant cost savings on procedures, compared to hospitals in the United States, and a higher, more personalized level of nursing care than Westerners are accustomed to receiving in hospitals back home. In 2005, one Bangkok hospital took in 150,000 treatment seekers from abroad. In 2006, medical tourism was projected to earn the country 36.4 billion baht. One patient who received a coronary artery bypass surgery at Bumrungrad International hospital in Bangkok said the operation cost him US$12,000, as opposed to the $100,000 he estimated the operation would have cost him at home in the US.

Hospitals in Thailand are a popular destination for other Asians. Another hospital that caters to medical tourists, Bangkok General Hospital, has a Japanese wing and Phyathai Hospitals Group has interpreters for over 22 languages, besides the English speaking medical staff. When Nepal Prime Minister Girija Prasad Koirala needed medical care in 2006, he went to Bangkok. While it is not commonly known outside Thailand, the modern Thai medical system had its origins in the United States when Prince Mahidol of Songla, the King's father, earned his MD degree from Harvard Medical School in the early 20th century. Prince Mahidol and another member of the Thai Royal Family paid for an American medical education for a group of Thai men and women. Prince Mahidol also convinced the Rockefeller Foundation to provide scholarships for Thai citizens to study medicine and nursing. Funds from the Rockefeller Foundation were also used to help build modern medical training facilities in Thailand. The men and women who studied medicine and nursing as a result of Prince Mahidol's efforts became the first educators for the modern Thai medical system.

Today many Thai physicians hold US professional certification. A number of Thai hospitals have relationships with facilities in the US. The US Consular information sheet gives the Thai healthcare system high marks for quality, particularly facilities in Bangkok. In Thailand, there is modern infrastructure, with clean, safe streets. According to the US Consular information sheets, the crime rate in Bangkok is lower than that of many US cities.

Personal safety is another factor to consider when traveling abroad both for vacation as well as healthcare. Thailand offers everything from cardiac surgery to organ transplants at a price much lower than the US or Europe, in a safe, clean environment. Thailand has long been a destination for medical tourists, and has a growing number of hospitals with JCAHO accreditation. Over one million people per year travel there for everything from cosmetic surgery to cutting edge cardiac treatment. Don Ho, the famous Hawaiian entertainer, recently received cutting-edge adult stem cell cardiac treatment at a Bangkok hospital. Six weeks later he had recovered sufficiently from his nonischemic cardiomyopathy and was able to return to the stage.

MEDICAL TRAVEL: RISKS AND REWARDS

Medical tourism does carry risks that local medical procedures do not. Should complications arise, patients might not be covered by insurance or be able to seek adequate compensation via malpractice lawsuits, though it should be noted that the malpractice insurance is a considerable portion of the cost in the West. For some living in remote rural areas, travel to another country is almost as expensive as travel to a large city in their own country.

Nations such as India or Thailand have different infectious diseases, and different prevalence of the same diseases, than home nations such as the US, Canada, UK. Exposure to foreign diseases without having built up natural immunity can be a hazard for weakened individuals, specifically for gastrointestinal diseases (e.g Hep A, amoebic dysentery, bacteria) which could weaken progress, mosquito transmitted diseases, and influenza, TB, etc. (75% of South Africans have latent TB) Also, travel soon after surgery can increase the risk of complications, as can vacation activities. For example, scars will be darker and more noticeable if they sunburn while healing. Long flights can be bad for those with heart (thrombosis) or breathing related problems (low oxygen environment), not to mention uncomfortable. However, because in poor tropical nations diseases run the gamut, doctors seem to be more open to the possibility of any disease, including HIV, TB, and typhoid, there are cases in the West where patients were consistently misdiagnosed for years because it is perceived to be "rare" in the West, a famous case of the misdiagnosis and death of a CDC researcher from TB, something that few would rule out in India or Thailand.

6

Indian Medical Tourism

AYURVEDA IN INDIA

Ayurveda in India—the science of life, the origin of most forms of natural and alternative medicine—has its mention in one of the oldest (about 6,000 years) philosophical texts of the world, the Rig Veda. The Sutrasthana of Charaka Samhita, a much referred ayurvedic text, says; "The three—body, mind and soul—are like a tripod, the world stand by their combination; in them everything abides. It is the subject matter of ayurveda for which the teachings of ayurveda have been revealed." (1.46-47)

In its broader scope, ayurveda in India has always sought to prepare mankind for the realization of the full potential of its self through a psychosomatic integration. A comprehensive health care is what this natural and alternative medicine prescribes for the ultimate self-realization. "Life (ayu) is the combination (samyoga) of body, senses, mind and reincarnating soul. Ayurveda is the most sacred science of life, beneficial to humans both in this world and the world beyond." —Charaka Samhita, Sutrasthana, 1.42-43.

The verses of Rig Veda, the earliest source of ayurveda, refer to panchamahabhut (five basic elements of the entire creation), and the three doshas or primary forces of prana or vata (air), agni or pitta (fire) and soma or kapha (water and earth) as comprising the basic principles of ayurveda. One branch of Indian philosophy—Sankhya states that there are 24 elements, all of which constitute the foundation of the gross world: earth, water, fire, air and ether. These five elements in different combinations constitute the three body types/doshas—vata dosha (air and ether), pitta dosha (fire) and kapha dosha (earth and water). The panchamahabhut and the dosha theories are the guiding factors of ayurveda as a therapeutic science. The Rig Veda also mentions organ transplants and herbal remedies called soma with properties of elixir. This science or knowledge of healing, as mentioned in the Rig Veda, was revealed to Rishi Bharadvaja from the great Cosmic Intelligence. The knowledge consists of three aspects known as the Tri-Sutras of ayurveda, which are—etiology or the science of the causes of disease, symptomatology or the study and interpretation of symptoms and medication and herbal remedies.

Approximately, during 4,000 to 3,000 BC, Sam Veda and Yajur Veda, the second and third Vedas came into being. Chanting of mantras and performance of rituals were, respectively, dealt in these two Vedas. And, during 3,000 to 2,000 BC Atharva the fourth Veda was authored, of which ayurveda is an upaveda (subsection). Though it had been practiced all along, it was around this time that ayurveda in India, was codified from the oral tradition to book form, as an independent science. It enlists eight branches/divisions of ayurveda: Kayachikitsa (Internal Medicine), Shalakya Tantra (surgery and treatment of head and neck, Ophthalmology and Otolaryngology), Shalya Tantra (Surgery), Agada Tantra (Toxicology), Bhuta Vidya (Psychiatry), Kaumarabhritya (Pediatrics), Rasayana (science of rejuvenation or anti-aging), and Vajikarana (the science of fertility). The oldest treatise available on this codified version is Atreya Samhita.

The most fascinating aspect of ayurveda is, it was using almost all methods of healing like lifestyle regimen, yoga, aroma, meditation, gems, amulets, herbs, diet, jyotishi (astrology), color and surgery etc. in treating patients. Though ayurveda came into being as an independent upaveda of Atharva Veda, it has close links with other Vedas also. The Yajur Veda, which recommends rituals to pacify the panchamahabhuts in a view to heal both the Cosmic Being and the individual soul, is related to ayurveda in its principles and regulations of lifestyle.

The upaveda called Dhanur Veda or the martial arts and ayurveda both refer to each other in the treatment of marmas or sensitive points in the body. Ayurveda recommends specific ayurvedic massages, exercises and bodywork for this purpose.

Around 15,00 BC ayurveda was delineated into to two distinct schools: Atreya—The School of Physicians, and Dhanvantari—The School of Surgeons. This made ayurveda a more systematically classified medical science, hereafter. Dhanvantari, who is considered to be a reincarnation of Lord Vishnu, was the guiding sage of ayurveda. He made this science of health and longevity popular and widely acceptable. In fact, these two schools of thought led to the writing of two major books on ayurveda—Charaka Samhita and Susruta Samhita.

These two Samhitas were written in the early part of 1000 BC. The great sage- physician Charaka authored Charaka Samhita revising and supplementing the text written by Atreya, which has remained the most referred ayurvedic text on internal medicine till date. Susruta, following the Dhanvantari School of Thought, wrote Susruta Samhita, comprising the knowledge about prosthetic surgery to replace limbs, cosmetic surgery, caesarian operations and even brain surgery. He is famed for his innovation of cosmetic surgery on nose or rhinoplasty. Around 500 AD, Vagbhatt compiled the third major treatise on ayurveda, Astanga Hridaya. It contained knowledge comprising the two schools of ayurveda.

From 500 AD to 1900 AD, sixteen major Nighantus or supplementary texts on ayurveda like Dhanvantari Bhavaprakasha, Raja and Shaligram among others were written incorporating new drugs, expansion in applications, discarding of old drugs and identification of substitutes. These texts mention about 1814 varieties of plants in vogue.

Evidences show that ayurveda had nurtured almost all the medical systems of the world. The Egyptians learnt about ayurveda long before the invasion of Alexander in the 4th century BC through their sea-trade with India. Greeks and Romans come to know about it after the famous invasion. The Unani form of medical tradition came out of this interaction. In the early part of the first millennium ayurveda spread to the East through Buddhism and greatly influenced the Tibetan and Chinese system of medicine and herbology. Around 323 BC, Nagarjuna, the great monastic of Mahayana Buddhism and an authority on ayurveda had written a review on Susruta Samhita. In 800 AD ayurveda was translated into Arabic. The two Islamic physicians Avicenna and Razi Serapion, who helped form the European tradition of medicine, strictly followed ayurveda. Even, Paracelsus, considered to be the father of the modern western medicine toed the line of ayurveda, as well.

In the postmodern age, the popularity of this vibrant tradition of ayurveda lies in its, subtle yet scientific, approach to heal a person in its totality. It aims, not only at healing the body, but also the mind and spirit, at one go. Its unique understanding of the similarities of natural law and the working of human body, as well as its holistic treatment methods, help it to strike a balance between the two. This gives ayurveda an edge over other healing systems. Perhaps that's the reason behind ayurveda being the longest unbroken medical tradition in the world, today.

Charaka Samhita is considered to be the most ancient and authoritative writing on ayurveda available today. It also explains the logic and philosophy on which this system of medicine is based. The detailed biography of the composer of this treatise—that is, sage Charaka—is not known to the posterity. Interestingly, it is not an original writing of a single person rather like all Vedic knowledge it is a continuation and renewal of that ancient knowledge system. In fact, Charaka had redacted the Agnivesa Samhita (an edited version of Atreya Samhita). The available form of Charaka Samhita was again worked upon by Drdhabala (living in about 400 AD) long after sage Charaka.

According to Charaka, science is dependent upon yukti—a quality of the intellect that enables it to perceive phenomena brought into existence by a multiplicity of causes. Thus, it's not surprising that much of the treatise of Charaka Samhita is in the form of a symposium wherein groups of ayurvedic scholars take up a series of topics for discussion. This gives indication that the science of ayurveda is a product of constant verification, fine-tuning and authentication by an active community of physicians. The samhita mentions about the gradual development of the fetus within the womb in minutes that equals the modern medical version in accuracy. The language is Sanskrit and is written in verse form. The style is in keeping with the Vedic oral tradition of conserving knowledge. The samhita contains 8,400 metrical verses.

Charaka followed the Atreya School of Physicians, which predominantly deals with treatments through internal and external application of medicine. Though the samhita contains all the theoretical knowledge of ayurveda it's focus is on healing the body, mind and soul of a patient in the minimum invasive manner that's Kayachikitsa. Hence, he placed great emphasis on the diagnostic part of the treatment. So much so that he classified everything from solar calendar to topography to the timing of the birth of a child. He identified eight stages of a disease from its inception to the culmination. Charaka also laid great emphasis on the timing and manner of the collection of medicinal plants.

Charaka sought to correct the element of fire or the digestive function in a body. It sought to alter the chemical processes in the cells by purification methods and medicinal application. From a greater perspective Charaka laid emphasis for health and longevity to strike a balance between one's corporeal and spiritual being. That is the reason why Charaka went so detail into the diagnosis of a disease's origin.

Susruta wrote his samhita, the most authentic text on the practice of ayurvedic surgery around the sixth century BC Susruta is, also, renowned as the father of plastic surgery. He represents the Dhanvantari School of surgeons. His samhita discussed in minute details on how to perform prosthetic surgery to replace limbs, cosmetic surgery on nose and on other parts of the body, cesarean operations, setting of compound fractures, and even brain surgery. Susruta's original work seems to have been revised and supplemented by Nagarjuna between the third and fourth centuries AD.

This branch of medicine is believed to have arisen in part from the exigencies of dealing with the effects of war. Epic

Ramayana, mentions remarkable feats of surgery having taken place in the past. We have reference to the transplantation of an eyeball and a head in epics. The style Susruta Samhita is both prose and poetry with poetry being the greater portion. This work, also, is said to be a redaction of oral material passed down verbally from generation to generation.

This work is unique in that it discusses blood in terms of the fourth doshic principle. This work is the first to enumerate and discuss the pitta subtypes. Susruta details about 125 surgical instruments used by him mostly made of stones,wood and other such natural materials. The Susruta Samhita presents many innovations in ayurvedic surgery. Use of shalaka—meaning foreign body (here, rods or a probe etc.) is mentioned by Susruta. Some of the classifications found in the Susruta Samhita are not even traced by the modern medical science. It described five types of pterygium, and the prognosis it made about glaucoma has not been improved since. In fact he is the first surgeon in medical history who systematically and elaborately dealt with anatomical structure of eye.

Susruta has discussed about 72 diseases of the eye. He has stipulated drug therapy for various types of conjunctivitis and glaucoma along with surgical procedures of the removal of cataract, pterygium, diseases of ear, nose and throat.

The Susruta Samhita, besides being the most authentic text on practice and theory of surgery, is also the most commonly quoted text on health.

Astanga Hridaya is accepted as the third major treatise on ayurveda. Around 500 AD, Vagbhatt compiled this samhita. It contained knowledge comprising the two schools of ayurveda—the school of surgery and the school of physicians.

There is another similar work called the Astanga Sangraha belonging to the same period. It is slightly bigger in size than the Astanga Hridaya, and is written in verse form whereas the later text was in prose form. It is believed either there are two works by a person or two persons with the same name. However, both the works came into being after the Charaka and Susruta Samhitas.

The Astanga Hridaya primarily deals with kayachikitsa besides, discussing in detail about various surgical treatments. The kapha subtypes are first listed and described in this samhita, completing exhaustive explanation of vata, pitta, kapha with their five subtypes.

Astanga Hridaya seems to emphasize on the physiological aspect of the body rather than the spiritual aspects of it like its counterparts—Charaka and Susruta Samhitas. Despite that, the quality and range of its discussions about ayurveda makes it a work to reckon with.

Ayurveda is a simple, practical science of life, the principles and practices of which evolved through many centuries. Ayurvedic science is based on eternal wisdom of people who acquired the knowledge from experience and meditation. Ayurvedic system is applicable universally to all those seeking harmony and peace. The Classical Ayurvedic texts discuss all forms of science like biology, toxicology and subjects like philosophy and theology.

Ayurveda has its own views about principles and philosophy of life. Ayurvedic system describes man as a universe within himself which is a child of the cosmic forces. His existence is inextricably intertwined to the total cosmic manifestation. The entire universe, as well as the body is made up of five basic elements. These elements are Earth, Water, Fire, Air and Space.

The word Ayurveda is composed of two sanskrit terms - Ayu meaning life and Veda meaning knowledge. Therefore Ayurveda means the knowledge of life or science of life. It is defined as the science, through which one can obtain knowledge about the useful and harmful ways of life, happy and miserable types of life, conditions that lead to the above types of life, as well as, the very nature of life.

According to Ayurvedic medicine, human body consists of three primary life forces or biological humors, which are Vatha, Pitha and Kapha. These three doshas are called the tridoshas. A balance among these life forces is essential for proper health. Any imbalance among the tridoshas causes a state of unhealthiness or disease. Ayurvedic system says that this imbalance is the effect of the constant reaction of the internal environment of body to the changes in external environment. It is only required that we bring back normalcy to the balance of these doshas, to bring back the state of healthiness. Other basic concepts of Ayurvedic system are the Saptha Dhathus (the bodily tissues), Srotas (Channals), Ama (toxins and filthy matter) and the trinity of life - body, mind and spiritual awareness.

The first step in the method of diagnosis in Ayurvedic form of medicine is to determine the constitution of the person. That means it is the patient who is diagnosed first and not the disease.

The same disease might appear in different forms in two persons because their constitution is different. Due to this variation in constitution the medicines and treatment may be different for two people with the same illness. This difference in treatment methods according to the constitution is essential to bring back the natural balance of the biological humors. The constitutional approach is the essence of the Ayurvedic system. Understanding ones constitution helps one to lead a life style that is most befitting his constitution, thus optimizing his health and creative potential.

According to Ayurvedic system, human body consists of three primary life forces or biological humors, which are Vatha, Pitha and Kapha. These three doshas are called the tridoshas. A balance among these life forces is essential for proper health. Any imbalance among the tridoshas causes a state of unhealthiness or disease. Ayurvedic treatment measures include internal medicine, external medicine, surgical treatment and psychotherapy.

Ayurvedic treatments can be classified under two groups - tonification and reduction. Reduction therapies decrease excesses in the body while tonification methods nurture insufficiency in the body. Reduction therapy has two parts called pacification and purification. Pacification is done with herbs, fasting, exercise, sunbathing and exposure to wind. Purification is a special form of therapy for elimination of the disease causing humors. The power of Ayurvedic elimination therapy is its system for guiding the toxins to their sites for elimination. It consist of five parts - The pancha karmas - cleaning enemas, nasal medication, Purgation, Emesis and blood letting. All these require preliminary Ayurvedic practises of oleation and sweating. Kerala a southern state of India, has developed its own Ayurvedic treatment modalities like Dhara, pizhichil, Navarakizhi, Elakizhi, Sirovasthi, Thalapothichil etc. which are highly effective in a number of diseases which include Motor neuron diseases, Arthritis of various kinds, skin diseases, heart diseases, peptic ulcer, Asthama, Peripheral vascular diseases and Gynecological disorders. Ayurvedic pharmacology is based upon the concepts of rasa, veerya and vipaka. A vast variety of plants, metals, minerals, animals, birds and even mud and sand are used as medicines in Ayurveda.

Knowledge about Ayurvedic type of medicine is divided into eight branches. The branches are:

1. Kaya chikilsa (general medicine),
2. Shalya (surgery),
3. Shalakya (ENT and Ophthalmology),
4. Graha (Psychotherapy),
5. Damshitra (toxicology),
6. Bala (Pediatrics and Gynecology),
7. Jara (rejuvenation) and
8. Vrishya (Aphrodisiacs).

Of the above the seventh one, that is rejuvenation therapy is a unique method which Ayurveda performs. Until death our body is engaged in a continuous struggle against the aging process. Hence the body is called Shareeram - something that degenerates.

TREATMENT

Ayurveda, the ancient traditional method of treatment involving combinations of herbal medicines, physical massages and various other forms of therapy, offers excellent remedies for many illnesses. Rajah Healthy Acres uses these methods of Ayurveda to treat ailments like Anxiety, Arthralgia, Asthma, Back pain, Diabetes, Disc Prolapse, Diseases of the eye, Dislocation, Dystonia, Hemiplegia, Hypertension, Impotence, Infertility, Miscarriage, Motor Neurone Disease, Multiple Sclerosis, Obesity, Peptic Ulcer, Peripheral Neuritis, Psoriasis and other skin diseases, Rheumatic Joint pains, Rheumatoid Arthritis etc.

Apart from treatment for these diseases Rajah Healthy Acres also offers therapy that rejuvenate the body and mind from the ills arising out of the frictions of everyday life.

The general types of Ayurvedic treatments offered are :

Uzhichil

Special Kerala type of massage done by two persons using medicated warm oils.

Improves blood circulation, strengthens muscles and joints, provides good sleep, improves the skin texture and sheen and nourishes the nerves. Suitable for healthy people also.

Elakizhi

This is a process of massaging the body with heated cloth bag filled with fried medicinal leaves like ricinus, calatropis, tarmarind etc. Done by three people.

Stimulates the nerves and helps to reduce pain. This is done in cases of Rheumatism, arthritis, paralysis, sciatica, spondylosis and nervous disorders.

Navarakizhi

The body is massaged with linen bags filled with cooked Navara rice, frequently warming it in a mixture of decoction and milk. Done by three people.

It is a cardinal treatment for diseases affecting the nervous system. Pain, rheumatism, emaciation of limbs, stroke, hypertension, sciatica, spondylosis etc. are the indications.

Podikizhi

A type of massage with cloth bags filled with herbal powder, which will be warmed frequently. Done by three people.

Effective for inflammatory joint problems and primary stage of hemiplegia.

Udvarthanam

This is the process of massaging the body with herbal powders in a reverse order. This is, from down to up. The treatment is mainly for obesity, cholesterol and certain rheumatic complaints.

Thalapothichil

The head is covered with Amla (Indian gooseberry) paste prepared in buttermilk or some decoctions suitable for the condition. The head is covered with a banana leaf.

Effective for dealing with stress, anxiety, sinusitis, chronic headache, sleep disorders and hair loss.

Dhanyamladhara

Four people, using special pots pour a warm acidic herbal fluid (dhanyamlam) all over patient's body. Helps to reduce inflammation and pain in many cases and is a method of sweating without using oils. Done in cases of arthritis, stroke, rheumatism etc.

Pizhichil

Using special pots, pouring warm medicated oil all over the body along with gentle massage by two people and three assisting them with collecting and warming the oil. Helpful for many types of multi joint problems and hemiplegia. It is strictly done for specific illnesses.

Sirodhara

Literally it means poring of a liquid on the forehead in a continuous stream. According to the type of liquid used, Sirodhara can be classified into three.

1. Thailadhara - Sirodara with medicated oil.
2. Thakradhara – Sirodhara with medicated buttermilk.
3. Ksheeradhara – Sirodhara with medicated milk.

According to the liquid used, the effect will be different. Thailadhara is good for various types of nervous disorders like hemiplegia, facial palsy etc. Thakaradhara is good for various skin diseases, sleeplessness, stress and insanity. And Ksheeradhara is good for making the head cool for insomania.

Sirovasthy

Warm oils are kept on the head inside a leather cap. Highly effective in cases of facial paralysis, headaches, spondylosis, hemiplegia etc.

Snehapanam

This involves internal administration of medicated ghee in daily increasing doses and strict restrictions on diet and activities. This is the primary preparation for all the panchakarmas. This is an internal Shehana (oleation) procedure. It is helpful in many cases like allergic asthma, psoriasis, eczema, low immunity, hyper acidity, peptic ulcer, digestive disorders and in all kinds of mental illnesses.

Kadeevasthy

A particular oil is kept over the affected part (usually the lower back) inside a boundary made of some herbal pastes.

Gives good results in all kinds of back pains and other spinal disorders. The same procedure when done on the chest is called Urovasthy.

Thalam

Oils or pastes are applied on the middle of the head and kept for one hour.

Helpful in alleviating insomnia, high blood pressure, stress and vatha predominant conditions.

Lepanam

Herbal pastes are applied over the affected parts.

Usually done to reduce swelling, pain or inflammation of the joints. Also used to treat some skin diseases.

Pichu

Cotton pieces soaked in warm medicated oils are applied on the affected parts. This cotton will be wet with warm oil frequently.

Effective pain relieving method for muscles and joints. It can be done on head also for some types of headaches and problem of sense organs.

Avagaham

After some oil applications, the patient will be seated in a tub full of hot herbal decoction suitable for patient's condition.

For the diseases of spinal cord, hip and lower back. Also helpful in gynaecological conditions.

Upanaham

A poultice containing herbal pastes with some acidic liquids which will be applied on the affected parts and covered with leaves of calotropis, ricinus etc. and on top with cotton cloth. This will be retained on position at least for 12 hours day or night.

For inflammatory joint pains which helps to reduce stiffness and improve mobility of the joints.

Nethratharpanam

Well melted and strained medicated ghee will be collected in a ridge made around the eyes with black gram paste. For refractive errors and degenerative diseases of the eyes.

Putapakam

Herbal juice mixed with goat's milk is collected around the eyes similarly as in netthra tharpanam.

Relieves tiredness of the eyes due to nethra tharpanam and to clear vision.

Nethradhara

Eye wash with special herbal decoctions, done by two persons.

For eye infections and to refresh the eyes.

Aschyothanam

Application of eye drops.

Helpful in conditions like various eye infections, cataract etc.

Mukhalepam

A herbal powder is mixed with cow's milk and applied on the face. It is kept for one hour and then washed. This is a herbal face pack.

This helps to remove wrinkles and black marks, improve the skin tone and imparts a special glow to the face. The powder is a special of the Rajah Ayurvedic hospitals under which Rajah Islands falls.

Ksheeradhoomam

Steaming the patients face and neck with medicated milk steams.

Most important treatment in facial paralysis, diseases of the sense organs etc.

PANCHAKARMA TREATMENTS

Vamanam

Medically induced vomiting. This is the cleansing process for the upper respiratory tract and upper digestive tract. Effective in Kapha rogas and some skin diseases like leukoderma etc.

Virechanam

Medically induced purgation which cleanses the lower digestive tract. Almost all types of skin diseases and chronic rheumatic problems will be relieved by this.

Nasyam

It involves the administration of medicines through the nose in the form of drops or powders. It is one of the Panchakarmas. Highly effective for all kinds of headaches, paralysis, depression, stress, pain around the neck and shoulders, eye diseases etc.

Snehavasthy

Medicated oil mixed with some herbal paste and salt, is administered through the anus. The quantity of material will be decided according ti the strength of the patient and disease.

One with the lowest dose of oil is called Mathravasthy. Beneficial in chronic nervous disorders, joint problems and skin diseases.

Kashayavasthy

Enema done with a mixture of honey, salt, herbal paste, herbal decoction and medicated oils. This will be preceded by one or two Snehavasthy according to the condition of the patient. Combination of Sneha and Kashaya vasthys are helpful in some chronic rheumatic problems. Urinary stones, nervous disorders and in some gynecological problems. Apart from these treatments certain special treatments are also offered at the center. The tranquil surroundings of Rajah Healthy Acres, with its vast expanse of land and thick greenery, tucked away in a pleasant country side, is most becoming for these revitalizing treatments to take affect.

Location

Comfortably tucked away at Kootanad, in Palakkad district of Kerala, the evergreen state in southern India, Rajah Healthy Acres, an ayurvedic health centre, is a nature lover's delight. Set amidst a majestic and peaceful landscape of hillocks, small valleys, medicinal trees and flora. Perfect locale to calm your mind. The nearest airports to the center are the Cochin, Calicut and Coimbatore airports. If the guests prefer we can arrange transportation from & to any of these airports or the Shornur, Pattambi, Kuttipuram and Trichur railway stations.

If you wish to travel by road, the route to take from Cochin side is Trichur --->Kunnamkulam. Follow the road from Kunnamkulam to Calicut for about 6 Kilometers and you will reach Perumpilavu. From Perumpilavu take the road to Pattambi. Go on this road up to Kootanad junction which is about 8 kilometers away from Perumpilavu and take the road to the left which is the road leading to Edappal. You will reach the Ayurveda health center after traveling on this road for about two kilometers from Kootanad junction. If you are travelling from Calicut side take the national highway up to Edappal and take a left turn from Edappal junction. You have to take a right turn from Padinnarangadi junction (about 7 kilometers from Edappal) for the Pattambi road (People tend to go straight from this junction instead of taking the right turn). The Ayurveda health center is about 5 kilometers away from this junction.

Rajah Healthy acres is an Ayurvedic health center in a lush country side - quiet and serene with facilities set in a 180 acre spread of thick greenery. Here, you can opt for different traditional treatments of Ayurveda in the snug comforts of modern facilities. A centrally located health center, well equipped with complete Ayurvedic health care system, run by experienced physicians will provide the healing touch. A gymnasium, indoor and outdoor games, a medicated pool, a small library furnished with books on a variety of topics and vast extracts of winding ways for long peaceful walks. Trips are also arranged to local tourist spots.

A bit of Indian culture depicted in the form of traditional arts like Ottamthullal, Bharathanatyam and Kuchipudi will be arranged for you if you prefer.

For patients, the doctor will decide a diet plan according to the person's disease, bodily requirements and the season. All cottages are provided with kitchenettes if you prefer to cook your own food. Currently broadband Internet is available at Rajah Healthy Acres through the machines of the centre. RHA is considering providing Internet through Wi-Fi so that the guests can access the Internet through their own computers.

A 1500 square feet cottage, with air-conditioned, bedroom and guest bedroom. The facilities in the cottage include a living room with telephone, a verandah, treatment rooms and a driver's room. Patients undergoing treatment for specific illnesses will be charged on a per day basis. The figures shown under the title "Charges per day" is applicable for persons registered for such treatments. Approximate charges for food and treatment, for people undergoing treatment for specific illnesses are also shown under the title "Charges per day".

All charges shown below are in US Dollars.

CHARGES PER DAY RENT FOR BOORJAPATHIRAM COTTAGE IN US$ APPROXIMATE TREATMENT & FOOD CHARGES US$ $ 208 $ 47

Patients undergoing rejuvenation therapy can opt for a package from the packages list shown below. Any person who are not undergoing any form of treatment and are accompanying the patients will be charged USD $14 per day. Doctors may advice additional treatment depending upon the condition of the patient, which may cost approximately USD $5 per day per person.

Additional person (mentioned below) means a person other than the person in whose name the quarters is registered and who is staying in the same quarters and undergoing treatment.

AYURVEDIC STUDIES

All ayurvedic studies conducted on herbal and holistic medicine in ancient India, followed from the fountainhead of the two principle ayurvedic schools. The School of Physicians (Atreya) and the School of Surgeons (Dhanvantari) epitomized the eight main areas of ayurvedic studies and specialization during ancient times. The details of these eight branches of this natural alternative medicine are present in the three ancient ayurvedic texts of: Charaka Samhita, Susruta Samhita and Astanga Hridaya. The word 'kaya' (body) not only refers to the gross body of a person but to the subtle body as well. This natural alternative medicine recognizes that the body of a person is the product of the constant psychosomatic interactions. The imbalances in the three doshas of vata-pitta-kapha occur sometimes by the mind and sometimes by the body's dhatu (tissues) and mala (toxin deposits). Hence, the kayachikitsa branch of this system of herbal and holistic medicine, delves deep into ascertaining the root cause of the illness. Then only a suitable treatment is recommended to bring back mind and body into balance. Though the prescription might give an impression that the treatment is meant for the physical body, these in fact have a strong impact on mind and soul of a person.

The Charaka Samhita is the most important scripture on kayachikitsa. It discussed the basic principles of treatment (mentioned above), various types of therapies and purification or detoxification methods i.e. panchakarma. But, its thrust area has been diagnosis of a disease. Detail account of various methods of diagnosis, study of various stages of symptoms and the comprehensive management of debilitating diseases like diabetes mellitus, tuberculosis, asthma and arthritic conditions. The section of Nidana Sthana of Charaka Samhita deals with etiology, pathogenesis and diagnosis of an illness. Six stages of the development of disease are enumerated as aggravation, accumulation, overflow, relocation, build up in a new site and manifestation into a recognizable disease (it is interesting to note that modern medical science can only detect a disease during the fifth or sixth stages of the illness). In kayachikitsa there is always an opportunity to stop the disease at each stage preventing its full manifestation.

One of the significant methods of treatment under kayachikitsa is panchakarma. This is a method of reversing the disease path from its manifestation stage back into to its site of original development through special forms of emesis, purgation and enema etc. Another unique aspect of kayachikitsa is rejuvenation called kaya kalpa. The term kaya kalpa means renewal of body. According to ayurveda the human body is made of seven types of dhatu or tissues-structures—plasma, blood, muscle, fat, bone, marrow and reproductive fluids. To prolong the youthfulness of the body kayachikitsa applies several physical and mental disciplinary methods with special medicinal preparations, to rebuild the body's cells and tissues after the initial process of detoxification, through panchakarma.

Contrary to the modern concepts surgery was pioneered by ayurveda in ancient India. It is a significant branch of ayurveda. The name of the sage-physician Susruta is synonymous with surgery. From his treatise Susruta Samhita we come to know that thousand of years ago sophisticated methods of surgery were practiced in India. The original text of Susruta discusses in detail about an exhaustive range of surgical methods including about how to deal with various types of tumors, internal and external injuries, fracture of bones, complications during pregnancy and delivery, and obstruction in intestinal loop. Susruta was the first surgeon to develop cosmetic surgery. His surgical treatment for trichiasis can be to some of the modern operative techniques used for this eye disease.

The use of various surgical instruments is also described in the Susruta Samhita for the treatment. The instruments described were made from stone, wood and other such natural materials.

Shalya Tantra was popular because this could give fast relief as compared to the slow process of recovery from medicines or herbs. Charaka the best-known physician of ayurvedic medicine also recommended for Shalya Tantra in treatment of certain diseases, which required immediate attention like hemorrhoids.

The long foreign rule in India and lack of promotion stalled the progress of ayurvedic surgery in the middle of the second millennium. This branch of ayurveda deals in details with the etiology, diagnosis, prognosis, prevention and treatment of diseases of head, ear, nose, eye and throat. The name of this branch was called Shalakya due to excessive use of 'Shalaka', which means a rod or probe. Though all the three main classics of ayurveda deals on this subject, Susruta Samhita describes more deeply about this branch. So much so that some of the classifications found in the Susruta Samhita are mot even traced by the modern medical science. It described five types of pterygium, and the prognosis it made about aveitis and glaucoma has not been improved since. In fact he is the first surgeon in medical history who systematically and elaborately dealt with anatomical structure of eye. Susruta has discussed about 72 diseases of the eye. He has stipulated drug therapy for various types of conjunctivitis and glaucoma along with surgical procedures of the removal of cataract, pterygium, diseases of ear, nose and throat besides cosmetic surgery for traumatized nose and ear (rhinoplasty and auraplasty).

Apart from these complicated methods of treatment the three samhitas—Charaka, Susruta and Astanga Hridaya, recommended simple home remedies for minor problems like dryness of eye, migraine and mouth ulcers etc. which are being successfully administered even today. Agada tantra or Toxicology branch of ayurveda described about various methods of cleaning the poisons out of the body as well as recommends antidotes for particular poisons. It deals with a wide range of natural toxins originating from wild lives (animals, birds, insects etc.), plants/herbs (belladonna, aconite etc.), vegetables, minerals (leads, mercury, arsenal etc.) and artificial poisons prepared from poisonous drugs. This branch also deals with air and water pollution, which are basically the causes of various dangerous epidemics.

The three samhitas described about this branch of toxicology, which also include description, and disadvantages of food of opposite qualities, drugs and food causing chronic poisoning symptoms. In ayurveda certain poisons are used as medicines after proper processing and quantification. Precious stones like diamond, ruby and poisonous minerals like lead and mercury were in use for this purpose.This branch also has information regarding fatal doses of various poisons, which are resorted to in a view to administer those into an enemy's body system.

This branch of kaumarabhritya deals comprehensively about prenatal, postnatal baby care and gynecology. With the view to achieve its ultimate aim of creating a healthy and disease free society ayurveda strives to make the baby from the time of its conception upto the time of its growth into an adult.

Kaumarabhritya has recognized that the mental and physical state of the mother has direct links with the health of the child. It has recommended particular diet, regimen, nutrition and conduct for women during and after delivery. So advanced was this science that thousands of years back Charaka described the growth and progress of fetus in minute detail. Even it mentioned about a technique called punsanvan vidhi for having a child of one's desired gender, intelligence and constitution. This branch meticulously dealt with the problem of infertility—its causes and treatment methods. Apart from that kaumarbhritya deals with various disorders concerning children's health such as gastrointestinal diseases, teething disorder, rickets other than midwifery. Ayurveda in this branch of science explains the art of producing healthy progeny for the creation of a better society. Hence, deals with various diseases like infertility and conditions relating to weak shukra dhatu or the vital reproductive fluids of the body. Apart from prescribing a lot of effective formulations to provide nutrition to enhance the quality of this vital body fluids it specifically emphasized to lead a highly disciplined life.

This branch of ayurveda highlighted that celibacy is essential for good health. It helps increase the will power, intellect and memory in addition to a healthy body. The shukra dhatu has a direct link with ojas or the immunity of the body. Hence, vajikaran prescribed the therapeutic use of various aphrodisiacs and tonic preparations for enhancing the vigor and reproductive capabilities of men that also strengthens other body tissues (dhatus) like muscles, fats, bones and blood. This branch of ayurveda specifically deals with the diseases of mind or psychic conditions, which can be caused by super natural forces. Different experts have explained the word bhuta differently. Some experts say that bhuta means ghosts and similar bad spirits who cause abnormal psychological conditions. Others say bhuta represents microscopic organisms such as virus, bacteria that are not visible to naked eye. Ayurveda also believes in the past karma as a causative factor of certain diseases. Bhuta Vidya deals with the causes, which are directly not visible and have no direct explanation in terms of tridosha.

In many cases illness is caused by the disturbance of mind, where rajas (passion) and tamas (ignorance) are supposed to be the contributing factors. These problems can be related to modern psychiatry.

Bhuta Vidya mention use of various disinfectant plants under the title of 'graha vidya dravya' for fumigation to make the atmosphere germ free. In addition to this herbs, diet, use of mantras and yogic therapies like meditation and pranayama to pacify the psychological disturbances of a patient. All therapies in ayurveda aim to provide good all round health, so that people can engage in achieving the real goal of life—self-realization. The rasayana therapy increases the life force (ojas) and immunity of a person and thus there is a regeneration of cells and tissues in the body. Rasayana is a therapeutic process to defer old age. The sages of ancient times led long, disease-free, and vigorous lives with the help of rasayanas. Lord Indra is supposed to have given the knowledge of these panaceas to the sages.

Literally, rasayana means the augmentation of rasa, the vital fluid produced by the digestion of food. It is the rasa flowing in the body which sustains life. Rasayana in ayurveda is, the method of treatment through which the rasa is maintained in the body. Another connotation of rasa in ayurveda is that it is a herbal medicine, which maintains the life and health of the individual, and increases his bodily and mental vigor. herbal medicines are categorized according to whether they promote general health and longevity, sexual vigor, immunity. The three medicine categories are known in ayurveda as rasayana, vajikarana, and aushadhis, respectively. These categories are complementary to each other. Rasayanas prepared from the herbs and medicinal plants of amalaki, haritiki, triphala, bhringaraja, ashwagandha, punarnava, chitraka and many other herbal medicines have been used from time immemorial and have been instrumental in giving long, disease-free, and vigorous lives to their users.

The human body contains some chemical elements, which are known as trace elements. Nine such elements are now recognized: cobalt, copper, fluorine, iodine, iron, manganese, molybdenum, selenium, and zinc. Ayurveda has always been using various metals, jewels, and pearls as medicines for certain deficiency diseases. These elements are turned into calxes or bhasmas for administration in different diseases. Calxes of gold, silver, copper and iron are widely used.

Jewels or ratnas include precious and semiprecious stones, which are used as drugs because of their therapeutic properties. Major jewels or maharatnas include: diamond—hiraka; ruby—manikya; pearl—mukta; topaz—pushparaga; sapphire—neelam; emerald—tarksha; cat's eye—vaidurya; zircon—gomedak; and caulk—vidruma. Uparatnas or minor jewels like sun-stone—suryakant , moonstone—chandrakanta, and crystal—sphatik were in use. The calx of diamond is a powerful cardiac tonic and one of the best elixirs. It was applied in curing diabetes, urinary troubles, and anemia. Because of its powerful aphrodisiac qualities the calx of diamond was used to treat impotence. The calx of rubies was used to increase intelligence, virility, and longevity. It also cures disorders produced by the vitiation of the three doshas. Much more than physical health, ayurveda begins with healing genetic physical weakness. It goes a great length to ascertain these inherited hindrances in one's being.

Then it recommends practice of suitable lifestyle regimens, which guard those faults, and use herbs and essential oils to heal and mend those weaknesses. Another aim of ayurvedic is to ensure balance of the three doshas. Following these rules the rasayana branch of treatment resorts to herb preparations and oils, bodywork, meditative practices, mantra exercises and breathing/pranayama to attain total mind-body healing. Rasayana oils have properties to bring balance in specific dosha types.

Administration of Rasayana

The Rasayana therapy is taken in two different ways:

Kutipravesika

In this process, elaborate arrangements are made for the construction of a special type of cottage where the individual is supposed to stay secluded, while taking the Rasayana. The person has to strictly follow the diets and other instructions of the physician. Here, he undergoes the detoxification process called Panchakarma therapy before taking the rejuvenation. Rejuvenation is done with help of some specific medicinal formulations and a specific lifestyle regimen. Kaya kalpa is a special rejuvenating method. The term kaya kalpa means renewal of body. According to ayurveda the human body is made of seven types of dhatu or tissues-structures such as plasma, blood, muscle, fat, bone, marrow and reproductive fluids. To prolong the youthfulness of the body several physical as well as mental disciplinary methods along with rasayanas or herbal medicines are used, to rebuild the body's cells and tissues after the initial process of detoxification—panchakarma. Kaya kalpa is that unique therapy, which brings about complete rejuvenation of the body through cell and tissue renewal. It is supposed to endow an individual with longevity, memory, intellect, youth, strength of sensory and motor organs, even, an excellent complexion and voice.

Vatatapika

This method is best for people who don't have time to stay in the ayurvedic clinic to take the first kind of rejuvenation. It comprises of different types ayurvedic herbal preparations which are taken as prescribed by the doctor. Rasayana is held as the culmination of ayurvedic wisdom.

Holistic Health

Ayurveda's focus on an individual's holistic health rather than merely the physical body, is the most beneficial aspect of ayurvedic medicine. It works on the principle that a perfect health condition is achievable through the psychosomatic integration in a person. Ayurveda provides us with a unique physical purification method called panchakarma and various ayurvedic herbal health remedies for mental and spiritual well-being. The ultimate goal of ayurveda is to create a state of holistic health for the individual, to create, consequently, a healthy society and environment with its herbal health remedies. To attain this state ayurveda believes one's life must move in harmony with nature's rhythms and its laws. Because, ayurvedic medicine recognizes the human body is part of nature, rather a microcosm of the universe. The five great elements of the universe forms the three doshas of the human body, and a balance among the three doshas is necessary for the perfect working of the whole mechanism of body, mind and soul.

These holistic health benefits of ayurveda encompasses the physical, mental as well as the spiritual aspects of a person.

According to ayurveda each individual is a combination of the three doshas of vata, pitta and kapha or one of these doshas. The basic constitution represents the individual's psychological and physical nature, distinctly. The tridoshas governs all metabolic activities in an individual. Within each person the doshas are adjusting to countless changes in the doshas of nature, in addition to the changes within one self. Noninvasive diagnostic ayurvedic treatments are beneficial for chronic patients suffering from diseases such as diabetes, heart ailments and cancer. Ayurvedic medicine resorts to outward diagnosis of symptoms by studying a patients' habits—diet and daily life, pulse, tongue, nail, face, lip, eye, nature of perspiration etc. Difficult diseases like asthma and tumor growths (gulmas) are managed effectively by these diagnostic methods.

Detoxification methods of ayurveda like panchakarma and other herbal health remedies, when applied wholly or singly, make the body more responsive to medicines and treatment. It hastens the healing process.

Various yogasanas prescribed by ayurveda help prevent the diseases from occuring and accumulating. Yogasanas achieve the twin purpose of strengthening body-parts such as bones, muscle and vital organs like heart, liver, stomach, intestine as well as keeping our blood circulation and psychological conditions strong and resilient.

Most importantly, a discerning diet according to one's dosha type, and well-regulated life (dinacharya) helps strengthen one's natural immune system.

Perhaps ayurveda is the first such medical systems who recognizes that all diseases are but the direct manifestation of one's mental conditions. It says human mind consists three states or trigunas—sattva, rajas and tamas. Any disturbances in the equilibrium of the tri-gunas, manifest in physical illness according to the intensity or nature of the disturbances. In fact, the condition of body and mind are integral to the overall health of an individual.

When the mind is stressed the stress hormone cortisone is released by adrenal glands. The level of hormone released affects the total volume of the brain's hippocampus, which regulates our memory. Stress also affects all our decision-making activities in every field of life. Ayurveda stresses on four principles—regulation in ahara (food habit), vihara (activities), nidra (sleeping habit), and maithuna (sexual habit), to maintain the balance and equanimity of the mind. Especially its guidelines for an intelligently regulated diet and daily routine are, now, accepted techniques for stress management. Ayurvedic massages, inhalation of herbal (Aromatherapy) preparations, panchakarma (nasya) besides the much-tested yogasanas and meditation leave a calming effect on the nerves.

According to ayurveda, tamasic (inertia, short of judgment) and rajasic (excessive activities, short of judgment) tendencies of mind prompt an individual to indulge in criminal or violent activities, telling lies and other such misconduct. This gives rise to negative thoughts like fear, anxieties, insecure feeling, greed, jealousy and anger.

Various advanced ayurvedic treatments were born out of a necessity to keep the mind and body in perfect shapes to pursue the path of self-realization. Each individual is believed to possess undefined measures of creative capability, which, ideally, need to be realized. To achieve this, ayurveda emphasizes that the individual has to experience its oneness with the universe. The balance of tri-doshas and tri-gunas is imperative in this regard, for the individual needs to remain in balance within itself and in harmony outside with the nature.

The treatment methods, diet and lifestyle regimen in ayurveda are meticulously planned to heal the body as well as enrich the mind and the soul of each different individual. So that each can improve from their own levels to the higher goal of realizing the full self-potential. It was with ayurveda that the unique longevity and rejuvenating method of rasayana was born for mankind to progress in the path of spirituality.

7

Development of Tourism in India

INTRODUCTION

Tourism development in India has passed through many phases. At Government level the development of tourist facilities was taken up in a planned manner in 1956 coinciding with the Second Five Year Plan. The approach has evolved from isolated planning of single unit facilities in the Second and Third Five Year Plans. The Sixth Plan marked the beginning of a new era when tourism began to be considered a major instrument for social integration and economic development.

But it was only after the 80's that tourism activity gained momentum. The Government took several significant steps. A National Policy on tourism was announced in 1982. Later in 1988, the National Committee on Tourism formulated a comprehensive plan for achieving a sustainable growth in tourism.

In 1992, a National Action Plan was prepared and in 1996 the National Strategy for Promotion of Tourism was drafted. In 1997, a draft new tourism policy in tune with the economic policies of the Government and the trends in tourism development was published for public debate. The draft policy is now under revision.

The proposed policy recognises the roles of Central and State governments, public sector undertakings and the private sector in the development of tourism. The need for involvement of Panchayati Raj institutions, local bodies, non-governmental organisations and the local youth in the creation of tourism facilities has also been recognised. The other major development that took place were the setting up of the India Tourism Development Corporation in 1966 to promote India as a tourist destination and the Tourism Finance Corporation in 1989 to finance tourism projects.

Altogether, 21 Government-run Hotel Management and Catering Technology Institutes and 14 Food Craft Institutes were also established for imparting specialised training in hoteliering and catering.

TOURIST ATTRACTIONS

India is a country known for its lavish treatment to all visitors, no matter where they come from. Its visitor-friendly traditions, varied life styles and cultural heritage and colourful fairs and festivals held abiding attractions for the tourists.

The other attractions include beautiful beaches, forests and wild life and landscapes for eco-tourism, snow, river and mountain peaks for adventure tourism, technological parks and science museums for science tourism; centres of pilgrimage for spiritual tourism; heritage trains and hotels for heritage tourism. Yoga, ayurveda and natural health resorts also attract tourists. The Indian handicrafts particularly, jewellery, carpets, leather goods, ivory and brass work are the main shopping items of foreign tourists. The estimates available through surveys indicate that nearly forty per cent of the tourist expenditure on shopping is spent on such items.

GROWTH

Domestic tourism is as old as the Indian society. According to available statistics, domestic tourism has grown substantially during the last one decade. It increased to 167 million in 1998 from just 64 million in 1990, thus registering a compound annual growth of 12.8 per cent.

The growth of inbound tourism since Independence has been quite impressive. It was just around 17 thousand in 1951. From this level it rose to 2.36 million in 1998. Tourism receipts on the other hand have grown at a phenomenal rate of 17 per cent to Rs.11,540 crore in 1998 from Rs.7.7 crore in 1951.

ECONOMIC IMPACT

Tourism has emerged as an instrument of employment generation, poverty alleviation and sustainable human development. During 1998-99, employment generation through tourism was estimated at 14.79 million.

Foreign exchange earnings from the tourism sector during 1998-99 were estimated at Rs.12,011 crore. Tourism has thus become the second largest net foreign exchange earner for the country.

Tourism also contributed Rs.24,241 crore during 1998-99 towards the country's Gross Domestic Product (GDP).

THRUST AREAS

In order to speed up the development of tourism in the country several thrust areas have been identified for accomplishment during the Ninth Five Year Plan (1997-2002). The important ones are development of infrastructure, products, trekking, winter sports, wildlife and beach resorts and streamlining of facilitation procedures at airports, human resource development and facilitating private sector participation in the growth of infrastructure.

ORGANISATION

The organisations involved in the development of tourism in India are the Ministry of Tourism with its 21 field offices within the country and 18 abroad, Indian Institute of Tourism and Travel Management, National Council for Hotel Management and Catering Technology, India Tourism Development Corporation, Indian Institute of Skiing and Mountaineering and the National Institute of Water Sports.

BOOSTING TOURISM

Some of the recent initiatives taken by the Government to boost tourism include grant of export house status to the tourism sector and incentives for promoting private investment in the form of Income Tax exemptions, interest subsidy and reduced import duty. The hotel and tourism-related industry has been declared a high priority industry for foreign investment which entails automatic approval of direct investment up to 51 per cent of foreign equity and allowing 100 per cent non-resident Indian investment and simplifying rules regarding the grant of approval to travel agents, tour operators and tourist transport operators.

CELEBRATIONS

During the Golden Jubilee celebrations of India as a Republic, the Ministry of Tourism made special efforts to publicise the tourism potential of India. The first-ever Indian Tourism Day was celebrated on January 25, 1998. Bauddha Mahotsav was organised from 24th October to 8th November 1998. The Year 1999 was celebrated as Explore India Millennium Year by presenting a spectacular tableau on the cultural heritage of India at the Republic Day Parade and organising India Tourism Expo in New Delhi and Khajuraho. The Wong La Millennium was held from April 1999 to January 2001. A special calendar of events has been formulated for highlighting contributions to Millennium events by various places in all the States. An official website of the Ministry of Tourism has also been created for facilitating dissemination of information on tourism.

CONSTRAINTS

The major constraint in the expansion of international tourist traffic to India is non-availability of adequate infrastructure including adequate air seat capacity, accessibility to tourist destinations, accommodation and trained manpower in sufficient number.

Poor visitor experience, particularly, due to inadequate infrastructural facilities, poor hygienic conditions and incidents of touting and harassment of tourists in some places are factors that contribute to poor visitor experience.

To sum up, Indian tourism has vast potential for generating employment and earning large sums of foreign exchange besides giving a fillip to the country's overall economic and social development. Much has been achieved by way of increasing air seat capacity, increasing trains and railway connectivity to important tourist destinations, four-laning of roads connecting important tourist centres and increasing availability of accommodation by adding heritage hotels to the hotel industry and encouraging paying guest accommodation. But much more remains to be done. Since tourism is a multi-dimensional activity, and basically a service industry, it would be necessary that all wings of the Central and State governments, private sector and voluntary organisations become active partners in the endeavour to attain sustainable growth in tourism if India is to become a world player in the tourist industry.

ECO TOURISM AND SUSTAINABLE DEVELOPMENT

The Draft Tourism Policy 1997 states that "in the context of economic liberalisation and globalisation being pursued by the country, the development policies of no sector can remain static." The policy further states that "the emergence of tourism as an important instrument for sustainable human development including poverty alleviation, employment generation, environmental regeneration and advancement of women and other disadvantaged groups in the country" requires support to realise these goals. India's tourism resources have always been considered immense, in a tourism audit. The geographical features are diverse, colourful and varied. The coastline offers opportunities for developing the best beaches in the world. There are a wealth of eco-systems including bio-sphere reserves, mangroves, coral reefs, deserts, mountains and forests as well as an equally wide range of flora and fauna.

The Policy further states that "international tourists visiting interiors of the country for reasons of purity of the environment and nature contributes to the development of these areas particularly backward regions". Thus Tourism "should also become a reason for better preservation and protection of our natural resources, environment and ecology". The policy recognises that sustained growth of tourism can give rise to conflicts. To ensure that the growth of tourism takes place along desired lines, certain guidelines have been framed: 1.to remove the constraint of the information gap.

1. To create a tourist product that is desirable and supported by an integrated infrastructure.
2. To involve all agencies, public, private and government, in tourism development.
3. To create synergy between departments and agencies that have to deliver the composite tourist product.
4. To use both the circuit and scheme approach so that peoples participation through panchayats, local bodies, NGO's, and youth organisations will create a greater awareness of tourism. The Central Government can thus concentrate on larger investment oriented projects.
5. To create direct access for destinations off the beaten track.
6. To diversify the product with new options like beach tourism, forests, wild life, landscapes and adventure tourism, farm and health tourism.
7. To ensure that the development does not exceed sustainable levels.
8. To develop the seven north-eastern states, the Himalayan region and Islands for tourism.
9. To maintain a balance between the negative and positive impacts of tourism through planning restrictions and through education of the people for conservation and development.

The strategy for development should take into consideration the carrying capacity, local aspirations and benefits likely to accrue to the community. In particular specific policies and guidelines for eco-tourism development and adventure tourism are to be formulated, primarily through a regulatory framework.

The Draft Guidelines have been approved at a State Ministers Conference and have been circulated to various trade and industry bodies. The guidelines draw a distinction between mass or resort tourism and nature or eco tourism, as the kind of tourism that has a lower impact on the environment and requires less infrastructural development. The Ministry hopes that the environment conscious international tourist will be made aware that India is taking steps to protect its ecology and environment.

Apart from the do's and don'ts, the guidelines are governed by a tourism management plan, the key elements of which are the protection of natural resources and a positive involvement of local communities, along with an optimum number of environmentally conscious visitors.

The principles of management are scientific planning, effective control and continuous monitoring, development of physical infrastructure, zoning and a Management plan for public use of natural sites. The management plan should establish standards for resort development, style and location of structures, waste disposal, treatment of sewage, control of litter, use of public spaces and fragile areas. The operational guidelines rely on sensitisation of all the role players and this programme is based on a self-regulated environmental code.

Area specific rather than universal development plans keeping in mind the unique character of the location and its economic and social environment are important. This would help the State Government to coordinate with the industry in managing visitors and their activities. NGO's working on socio-economic programmes in forest and remote areas could have a closer coordination with tourism service operators to transfer economic benefits, particularly the handicraft production and marketing sector.

The guidelines are only a beginning, and it is hoped that with increasing awareness of the visitor the industry will regulate its practices. There is an emphasis on the needs and perceptions of the international tourist running through the discussion on the guide lines although the data from the National Parks makes it evident that the domestic tourists outnumber international visitors, although they do not pay the same amount as the foreign visitor either in entry fees or for board and lodging and transport facilities.

They do however demand a much higher per capita use of resources like water, fuel for heating and cooking and transport. They also make the same intensive use of time and try to maximize their stay by the number of animals and birds they can view in the 24-hour period.

It is interesting to note that no democratic participation has been called for in the policy formulation process, and all the amendments to the policy have come from trade associations and government think tanks. The tourism Advisory Committee also consists of eminent persons and community representation has been ignored. The elite nature of the policy makers is well represented in the quotations given above from the policy document.

The policy clearly recognises the debate on the tourism issue which has surfaced wherever tourism development, particularly in the case of tourism projects relating to the "gifts of nature" like beaches, rivers, mountains and forests, have already been developed. However, mere recognition of the hostility of people to tourism development is not enough to change the nature of tourism development or the resistance to tourism or what many have termed a poor tourism culture. Perhaps to understand this in a better perspective, we should look at the issue of sustainable development in a critical way. Perhaps we can question the impact of sustainable development on the environment and sift through the jargon of development planners, international agencies, and environmental activists to see how sustainable development can be achieved without all the contradictions that are apparent as in the case of the tourism sector.

Phrase SUSTAINABLE DEVELOPMENT Concepts Sustainability Development Connotations Literal, ecological, Social Process Objectives Meaning sustains sustains sustains growth/ anything, ecological social basis change basic needs basis of of human human life life conditions ecological social conditions conditions interpretations SD sustaining growth SD achieving traditional objectives + ecological and social sustainability (contradictory, trivial) (mainstream, meaningful) Semantic Map Sustainable development has become the developmental paradigm of the nineties but it remains a fashionable phrase that everyone pays homage to but no one cares to define. (Tolba, 1984).

To some extent the value of the phrase lies in its ambiguity. It allows people with irreconcilable positions in the environmental debate to appear to have found common ground without having to compromise their positions. The absence of semantic and conceptual clarity hampers a real debate. S. M. Lele (1991) has attempted a semantic map of Sustainable Development, which will help us to understand some of the positions in the debate. Is sustainable development ecologically sustainable and environmentally sound or is it a process of change that has sustainability added to it? Is it to be understood as sustained growth or successful development? Literally sustainable development is change that can be sustained or continued for the time period concerned. Development we can say with some confidence is a process of directed change, but any process embodies both the objectives and the means of achieving the stated objectives.

Objectives

Can we set sustainable objectives (as growth in sustained consumption of) for resources that now are recognised to have ultimate limits or what we may call non-renewable resources or what we may call the balance between the use and conservation of such resources? Even where we are concerned with socio-economic change, the discussion is not meaningful unless we state the objectives of change and why we should be concerned with continuing the process of change indefinitely. Is the change so envisaged to be broadly understood as social welfare? Can the increase in welfare continue indefinitely, and what will be its cost? Even where welfare is based on beneficiary oriented design (grass roots participation) as a procedural imperative, it tells us nothing about the overall goal of the developmental process since the beneficiaries need not conserve resources to achieve their welfare. The concept of sustainability originated in the context of renewable resources like forests and fisheries and was subsequently adopted by the environmental movement. In most cases it is understood to mean "the existence of the ecological conditions necessary to support human life at a specific level of well being through future generations." However, in addition to ecological conditions there are social conditions that influence ecological sustainability in a nature-people interaction. The social connotations have been described by Barbier (1987) who has defined social sustainability as "the ability to maintain desired social values, traditions, institutions, cultures or other social characteristics."

The term sustainability came into usage in 1980 when the IUCN presented the World Conservation Strategy where sustainable development was linked to conservation of living resources. However, the fundamental goals have often been lost sight of because of operational goals (e.g. food, water, shelter, health are fundamental goals to be realised through self reliance, cost effectiveness, appropriate technology, people centred-ness etc.) Consequently, the WCED made its definition brief: Social Development is development that meets the needs of the present without compromising the ability of future generations to meet their own needs. They did not make any assumptions on the direction in which changes in demand would take place. (E.g. equity, social justice, self-determination, or cultural diversity). India's tourism policy follows the mainstream SD thinking by adopting all the critical objectives: revive growth change the quality of growth meet essential needs for jobs, food, energy, water and sanitation ensure sustainable levels of population conserve and enhance the resource base reorient technology and management risk merge environment and economics in decision making reorient international economic relations make development more participatory.

These objectives are responsible for building a very broad consensus on the issue of sustainable development, yet the debate at the operational level continues. Most participants in the debate now accept that many human activities are reducing the long-term ability of the natural environment to provide goods and services, which will eventually affect human health and well being. Many also accept that poverty is devastating the lives of millions in the Third World since there is no consensus between what is environmentally necessary and what is economically and developmentally feasible. The level of interdependence between the two insights is yet to be incorporated in the concept of Social Development. Some problem areas are: Environmental degradation, already affecting millions in the Third World, is likely to reduce human well being across the globe. Who is responsible for this rapid degeneration? Is it the poor or the rich?

The poor have no option but to exploit resources for short-term survival. If we take the example of forests and their resources, which have been traditionally outside the market system and in the sphere of tribal or indigenous peoples rights, they are today seen as exploiters of the forests as against tourists, with all their demand for infrastructure and superstructure, who are seen to be conservationists. The interlinked nature of the problem of sustainability is such that the impact of degradation will be quicker on the poor than on the rich. Can Sustainable Development be the metafix it claims to be in reconciling increasing industrial, agricultural and resource use productivity with environmental needs.

The weakness of the Social Development argument lies in the techno-economic approach to solutions with regard to common property resource management, through know how transfers, resource pricing, subsidy policies and building management capabilities. (World Bank, 1987) Deeper processes such as land reforms, industrial demands on raw materials, over consumption, changing legal and political structures are either ignored or looked at in a cursory manner.

For instance how can we claim a consensus between those who are concerned for the survival of future generations with those who are concerned with the survival of wild life, or human health and subsistence? Unless we can identify the trade-offs necessary for each specific objective of sustainability, we will not have clarity in the discussion. We will also fail to understand why, even when there is a broad consensus, projects on the ground result in conflicts.

Suggested refinements could be: a distinction between ecological and social sustainability and in the process an identification of the inter-linkages a distinction between renewable and non-renewable resources, between environmental processes crucial to human life and crucial to other forms of life dependent on the resources, a distinction between the techno-economic aspects of social sustainability (infrastructure, services, government) with political and cultural sustainability, a distinction between equitable development and local participation, and decentralisation, what many have called NGOisation of sustainable development.

This is because no rigorous testing of local participation leading to social equity or to sustainable resource use have been reported. Case studies reflect personal, organisational or political preferences.

Tourism is one of the activities which has caused concern because of the effects of increasing human traffic on fragile environments. Countries which are looking towards Tourism as a means of economic growth, like India, have limited resources and cultural restraints and they have the greatest need to pay heed to the possible negative impacts of tourism.

Environmental Impact

The environmental impact of tourism is a basic issue, whether we are looking at a developed or an underdeveloped area, region or country. The costs of tourism for a country like India include extensive investment in fixed assets with a low rate of return for infrastructure, transportation, accommodation, cultural institutions, exhibition centres, and park facilities.

To this maybe added the social and cultural costs like additional demands on infrastructure like land, water, health services; the creation of new jobs for displaced people; the cost of positive community relationships; the disparity between the lifestyle of visitors and those who serve them; the possible friction between local residents and new users of valued local resources; the perception of local residents of the spending of scarce capital resources on what they consider low priority areas like tourism; cultural cost of alterations in local ceremonial or traditional values; loss of privacy for local communities as tourists come to gape at their living conditions and rituals.

Tourism also causes increasing congestion and pollution as thousands of visitors flock to parks and sanctuaries in motorised vehicles; there are changes in accessibility, landscape and the ecological balance between man and nature; there is the cost, both monetary and human, of creating conservation zones (core/buffer) with unforeseen or undesirable side effects; which have been observed in the ecotourism movement.

The benefit of revenue from tourism does not always redress these problems but goes towards the cost of administering the project. The tourism industry is generally self-centred and not given to educational, cultural or exchange programmes on a philanthropic basis.

The natural environment, with the best will in the world, cannot escape damage with the volume of visitors. As more and more tourists, both domestic and international seek the exotic and remote destinations around the world, the likelihood of the environment suffering as a result become greater. Forests can suffer from trampling, fires, tree felling for facilities and waste. Wildlife, despite the protection in national parks, has suffered a loss of habitat, hunting and poaching, viewing and photographing, leading to an interruption of feeding and breeding patterns or hunting for food undisturbed. These are the prized moments for the viewer.

The trade in wild life trophies or tourist souvenirs is the more deliberately destructive aspect of such tourism. The building of tourist lodges in materials that are not integrated with the environment and the pressure they put on the land and water bodies is also wilfully destructive. Management techniques that include being less user friendly or control of numbers by closing access or by multiplying the number of attractions and areas or charging higher admission fees are generally not popular with the tourist or the tour operator and are also difficult to implement because of high administrative costs.

CONCLUSION

EQUATIONS, through its involvement in the field have had a variety of experiences relating to the debate on eco tourism and sustainable development.

The major issues that have emerged after the policy of notification of wild life sanctuaries and their management by the Forest Departments are quite disturbing. Wherever notification has led to displacement of people the experience of rehabilitation has not been successful and the conservation aims have not been met. Several sanctuaries have witnessed militant action by displaced communities against the developers of tourism.

In many cases the tourism aims have also not been met in making the sanctuary accessible to viewers, naturalists, wild life photographers. Tourism has not been able to counteract poaching and the most extensive and the oldest conservation project, Project Tiger has not been able to save the tiger population.

The commercialisation of the experience, like the privileging of one species, for example the tiger, has led to congestion and noise pollution and this has put a pressure on the management of the sanctuary to organise tiger shows which are putting a pressure on the feeding and mating habits of the tiger. These are very invasive techniques of experiencing the wild.

On the plus side, the concept of beneficiary led development has helped indigenous people to organise against their displacement and exploitation as well as to fight for the retention of their traditional rights and life styles. Environmentalists have not only been involved in such organisations and movements but have done valuable documentation. This has influenced many urban visitors to be more sensitive to the wild and to follow the rules when participating in eco-tourism. This has also led to the development of a code of conduct for the tourist, the industry and the administrator. These attempts are in a very nascent stage. The kind of co-ordination that is required between the environmentalist and economist is just beginning to emerge and have still to counter the myths of neo-classical economists in the field of tourism. But a beginning has been made.

8

Indian Policy of Tourism

INTRODUCTION

The objective of this report is to assess the impact of Tourism Policy on the tourism sector and make a preliminary study of the possible impact such policy imperatives might have on the socio-economic fabric of the country.

The study, commissioned by EQUATIONS, Bangalore, utilised a methodology involving a historical preview of the evolution of Tourism Policy since 1982, and an exploratory assessment of the impact. The study material included documentation available at EQUATIONS and relevant publications of the Union Government.

The impact assessment of the sectoral policies on the specified sector suffers from a serious methodological problem. Briefly, it may be argued that the development of a sector is not solely dependent on the factors within the sector: it is influenced by the general socio-economic environment, the political system and the overall policy framework.

Thus the study integrates within itself the dynamic aspects of historical changes that are taking place at the macro-economic level. Similarly, Tourism Policy would not have evolved on its own without being influenced by the general tenor of macro-economic policy. Tourism policy thus has a socio-political grounding as much as it has a macro-economic colouring.

The 1980s witnessed the era of liberalisation initiated by the Congress Government at the Centre. The process of liberating the Indian economy from the shibboleths of 'license-permit Raj' culminated in the initiation of the structural adjustment programme in 1992. "Objectives, Thrusts and Macro-economic Dimensions of the Eighth Plan" endorsed by the National Development Council, clearly outlines the context within which the structural reforms were initiated: "The need to restructure our systems of economic management has become an imperative if India is to emerge as a vibrant and internationally competitive economy in the 90's. Systems of control and regulation, developed for good reasons in the past have outlived their utility and some positively (sic) stand in the way of further progress. Such dysfunctional systems have to be overhauled in the light of emerging realities.

" The process of structural adjustments has brought about far reaching changes in the Indian economy at a breath-taking pace. The impact of these changes over the tourism sector need to be studied in a dynamic context. Nevertheless, the above should not be taken as ignoring the fact that sectoral policy does have a direct and unambiguous impact over the concerned sector.

Tourism Policy, as a statement of intent by the Government, would form the reference point for action and criticism. Any initiative by Government in Tourism by way of legislation or direct investment is envisaged within the framework of Tourism Policy. The debates in Parliament had taken recourse to the received policy of the Union Government while making references to particular cases. The backdrop of a policy always serves as a guideline for further executive and legislative initiatives. It would be cynical to regard these policy statements as mere exercises in eloquence and additions to the already existing volumes of wishful thinking.

Furthermore, Policy statements by Government should be viewed in their evolutionary stance. It would be a negation of the democratic content of our political system to view a Policy statement as a static and rigid formulation, at a point in time, applicable for years to come. Thus, since 1982, various initiatives undertaken by the Government need to be perceived as additions or modifications to the received Policy. While it may be argued that these changes in the policy are only marginal and superficial from the viewpoint of equity and social justice, it would be an oversimplification to view the latest policy statement as nothing but the "nth" version of the Policy formulated in 1982. Recognising the all-pervading inertia that looms large in matters governmental, one is often tempted to deny the scope for lobbying which makes possible the desired modifications in the policy corpus. In short, policy, as a body incorporating proactive intentions, is amenable to periodic reviews and possible modifications.

The issues stressed in the preceding paragraphs provide the framework within which Tourism Policy needs to be considered. In brief, there is more to policy in tourism than is found in the Tourism Policy. Perhaps, the links within a macro-economic framework need no special mention.

MAJOR POLICY INITIATIVES

The first ever Tourism Policy was announced by the Government of India in November 1982. It took ten long years for the Government to feel the need to come up with a possible improvement over this. Thus the National Action Plan for Tourism was announced in May 1992. Between these two policy statements, various legislative and executive measures were brought about. In particular, the report of the National Committee on Tourism, submitted in 1988 needs special mention. In addition, two five-year plans-the Seventh and the Eighth-provided the basic perspective framework for operational initiatives.

The Seventh Plan advocated a two-pronged thrust in the area of development of tourism, viz., to vigorously promote domestic tourism and to diversify overseas tourism in India. While laying stress on creation of beach resorts, conducting of conventions, conferences, winter sports and trekking, the overall intention was to diversify options available for foreign tourists. The Tourism Policy, 1982 was more an aggressive statement in marketing than a perspective plan for development. Its main thrust was aimed at presenting India to the foreigners as the ultimate holiday resort. With a view to reach this destination, the following measures were suggested by the Policy:

1. To take full advantage of the national heritage in arriving at a popular campaign for attracting tourists;
2. To promote tourist resorts and make India a destination of holiday resorts;
3. To grant the status of an export industry to tourism;
4. To adopt a selective approach to develop few tourist circuits; and,
5. To invite private sector participation into the sector.

The Planning Commission recognised tourism as an industry by June 1982. However, it took ten years to make most of the States to fall in line and accord the same status within their legislative framework. At the beginning of the Eighth Plan (1992-97), 15 States and 3 Union Territories had declared tourism as an industry. Four States had declared hotels as an industry.

The National Committee on Tourism was set up in July 1986 by the Planning Commission to prepare a perspective plan for the sector. Within the broad framework of the Seventh Plan, the Committee had to evolve a perspective plan for the coming years.

The Committee, headed by Mr. Mohammed Yunus, submitted its recommendations in November 1987. The list of Members was as impressive Mr. S.K. Mishra (Secretary, Department of Tourism), Mrs. Kapila Vatsayan, Mr. K.L. Thapar, Mr. Rajan Jaitley, Mr. A.B. Kerker, Mr. R.K. Puri and Mr Pran Seth. The Committee in its Report recommended that the existing Department of Tourism be replaced by a National Tourism Board. It suggested that there be a separate cadre of Indian Tourism Service to look after the functioning of the Board. It also submitted proposals for partial privatisation of the two airlines owned by the Union Government.

By September, 1987, the Central Government declared more concessions for the sector: these included tax exemption on foreign exchange earnings from tourism (a 50% reduction on rupee earnings and a 100% reduction on earnings in dollars), a drastic reduction in tariff on import of capital goods, and concessional finance at the rate of 1 to 5% per annum. The Tourism Development Finance Corporation was set up in 1987 with a corpus fund of Rs. 100 crores. Until then, the sector was financed on commercial lines by the Industrial Development Bank of India, Industrial Credit and Investment Corporation of India and other commercial banks.

The National Action Plan for Tourism, published in May 1992, and tabled in the Lok Sabha on 5 May 1992, charts 7 objectives as central concerns of the Ministry:

- socio-economic development of areas;
- increasing employment opportunities;
- developing domestic tourism for the budget category;
- preserving national heritage and environment;
- development of international tourism;
- diversification of the tourism product.,
- and, increase in India's share in world tourism (from the present 0.4% to 1% during next 5 years)

As per the Action Plan, foreign exchange earnings are estimated to increase from Rs.10,000 crores in 1992 to Rs.24,000 crores by 2000 AD. Simultaneously, the Plan aims at increasing employment in tourism to 28 million from the present 14 million. Hotel accommodation is to be increased from 44,400 rooms to 1,20,000 by 3 years. Other provisions in the Action Plan include a discontinuance of subsidies to star hotels, encouraging foreign investment in tourism and the setting up of a convention city for developing convention tourism.

The Action Plan envisages the development of Special Tourism Areas on lines of export processing zones. Special Central assistance is to be provided for the States to improve the infrastructural facilities at pilgrimage places. It proposes to set up a National Culinary Institute, and projects a liberalised framework for recognition of travel agents and tour operators.

The Eighth Plan document makes a special mention that the future expansion of tourism should be achieved mainly by private sector participation. The thrust areas as enumerated in the Plan include development of selected tourist places, diversification from cultural related tourism to holiday and leisure tourism, development of trekking, winter sports, wildlife and beach resort tourism, exploring new source markets, restoration of national heritage projects, launching of national image building, providing inexpensive accommodation in different tourist centres, improving service efficiency in public sector corporations and streamlining of facilitation procedures at airports.

The Eighth Plan aims at luring the high spending tourists from Europe and USA. It also envisages a 'master plan' to integrate area plans with development of tourism. This is envisaged to ensure employment opportunities for the local population.

In April 1993, the Government announced further measures aimed at export promotion. The existing Export Promotion of Capital Goods Scheme (EPCG) was extended to tourism and related services. Against the existing 35%, the tourism sector would now pay an excise duty of 15% only on capital goods import, subject to an export obligation of 4 times the cargo, insurance and freight (CIF) value of imports. With an obligation period of five years, this came as a boon to the hotel industry. The cost of construction had also come down by 20%.

In addition to the above policy pronouncements by the Union Government, our planners had envisaged the possibilities of developing specific regions on a zonal plank. Special area programmes like the Hill Area Development Programme and the Western Ghats Development Programme form part of the overall national plan.

The Eighth Plan document stipulates that the strategy in such designated special areas is to devise suitable location-specific solutions, so as to reverse the process of degradation of natural resources and ensure sustainable development. This approach perhaps needs to be integrated into the project of special tourism areas, now being made popular by the Government. Administrative Control and Developmental Compromises.

The federal principles enshrined in the Indian Constitution require that the tourism sector be treated as a State subject. As such, the Department of Tourism (under the Ministry of Civil Aviation and Tourism at the Centre) undertakes certain promotional and developmental activities with a view to enhance the sectoral potential. The Department has certain regulatory functions to perform involving the hotel industry, travel agencies and tourist operators.

Over the years, there has been considerable erosion of powers so far as State Governments are concerned. The sustained campaign for privatisation in all the policy documents has left limited space of operation for the States. The public sector is increasingly being perceived as an agent of inertia than of change and hence the pressure for a hands-off policy. On the other hand, the Union Government has been usurping the powers of the State with some pretext or the other. Promotion schemes, designed at the Centre, are transferred for implementation at the State level.

The special Central Assistance, for example, granted for the development of infrastructure at the pilgrim centres, carries with it a pre-defined scheme and mode of execution. Furthermore, there are occasions when the Centre forces the State Governments to extend certain subsidies and concessions to the sector. The terms of such concessions would have been fixed by the Centre and the States would have no choice but to fall in line.

For example, during the State tourism minister's conference in December 1991, the States were urged to freeze water and electricity rates for 10 years. They were also asked to exempt certain hotels from local and state taxes for 10 years. Seventeen circuits and destinations were identified under the National Action Plan for development through Central assistance and investment by the States and the private sector. The centres were identified by the Centre and the States were asked to do the needful. There were also times when the federal division of power resulted in operational contradictions.

For instance, by 1989, many foreign hotel chains like Hilton, Hyatt, Penta and Kempinski had applied for licenses for investing in India. However, the revenue departments of the respective States failed to locate and allocate land for the construction of hotels.

The scheme, thus, fell flat. Curiously, the Union Government was not hesitant to make use of Constitutional provisions when it suited its interests. As has been stated earlier, the Yunus Committee had suggested the creation of the Tourism Board on lines of the existing Railway Board. (Perhaps, it was the brainchild of Mr. K.L. Thapar, then adviser to the Planning Commission, in charge of Transport and Tourism Sector. Being from the Railway Service, it is not surprising that Thapar thought about a 'Tourism Board'). To begin with, the empowered committee of secretaries challenged the idea of creation of a Board. It was said that the Railway Board as an independent entity was created for historical reasons. It would be difficult for tourism to be looked after by a Board, because legally the sector would come under the Industrial (Development) Act. It was also found that such a Board would not be viable financially. In 1991, the think-tank on tourism created by Minister Madhavarao Scindia rejected the idea of a Board in toto. It was emphasised that the Board cannot be in charge of a sector that is basically under the jurisdiction of the States! Scope for Federal Interventions The previous section highlights the dubious ways by which the Centre attempts to hijack initiatives at the State-level. This is achieved essentially by threatening to curtail Central assistance or by cajoling through promises of more financial aid.

It is common knowledge that the resource-base of the States is very narrow, making them vulnerable at the negotiating table. However, States have the freedom to resist the Centre's strong-arm tactics, provided State assemblies stand-by the interests of the States. For instance, State legislatures may refuse to freeze water and electricity rates on grounds of revenue generation.

In that event, the concerned Chief Minister or the Minister of Tourism may convey the intensity of resistance that he is confronted with, and thus refuse to comply with the Centre's diktats. It is heartening to realise that the States have often exercised their power of self-determination and consequently refused to toe the line drawn by the Centre. This offers enough scope for possible interventions at the federal strata of our political system in matters of policy formulation. Privatisation and its Implications According to the Approach Paper to the Seventh Plan, " there is a vast potential for development of tourism in the country.

Tourism should be accorded the status of an industry. Private sector investment will have to be encouraged in developing tourism and public sector investments should be focused only on development of support infrastructure". Thus the seeds of private initiatives were sown during the Seventh Plan. The Government took the matter of privatising the tourism sector seriously by 1988. It was during the tenure of Mr. S.K. Mishra as Tourism Secretary that the talk of inviting private investment into the sector began.

The Government permitted foreign equity participation up to 5 1 %in tourism projects. Foreign charters were allowed to operate in the country for the first time. Foreign companies were allowed to repatriate their profits to the extent of 3%. The structural adjustment programme, initiated in June, 1992, paved the way for privatisation in almost all sectors of the economy. The Annual Plan (1992-93) document emphatically enunciated the Government's position vis-a-vis tourism: "(T)he future growth of tourism will have to be achieved mainly through private initiative.

The State will contribute to tourism by planning broad strategy of development, provision of monetary and fiscal incentives to catalyse private sector investment." The process of privatisation brought in its wake big investments and private involvement at various levels. As an offshoot, environmental considerations were thrown to the winds and there were instances of large scale human rights violation. The self-correcting nature of policy made provisions for stricter controls in this regard. More seriously, privatisation meant alienation of the majority of our population and their deprivation. Employment generated in tourism is generally seasonal and ill paid. The private sector-induced pockets of tourism had the potential of turning into centres of pollution, drug trafficking and prostitution. Industry Status Granted to Tourism The Seventh Plan proposed that tourism be declared an industry. However, it took time for the States to implement this, even though they agreed in principle.

The smokeless industry had the advantage of generating maximum value-added, because of low-cost inputs. The Tourism Policy Statement carried certain provisions in favour of the hotel industry. It stated that there should be provision for depreciation in the balance sheets of hotels. Being an export industry, hotels were to be given excise concessions. The provisions of the Monopolies and Restrictive Trade Practices (MRTP) Act were relaxed for hotels, because any hotel with 300 or more rooms would have incurred an investment of Rs. 25 crores. The document also hinted at lower tariffs for power and water and regulations for easy import of equipment. As a follow-up, hotel and shipping were added to the list of 27 industries exempted from Section 22 A of the MRTP Act. The consequences of declaring tourism as an industry need to be studied in detail. It is not possible to capture its implications in an exploratory work like this. However, it is obvious that the private sector has primarily benefited to a great extent by this measure. Importing Modifications to Policies We have earlier stated that the arena of policy formulation should be self-evaluating and self-correcting. In the case of Tourism Policy, this has proved to be the plus point.

As an illustration, the Policy statement of 1982 made no mention of infrastructure development. The successive governments at the Centre failed to create proper tourism infrastructure, thus resulting in loss of traffic. This lacuna was corrected in the National Action Plan. However, much of this change was due to intensive lobbying by such agencies like the Indian Association of Tour Operators (IATO), the Travel agents Association of India (TAAI) and the Indian Hotels and Restaurants Association (IHRA). It is for the voluntary agencies and pro-people forces to exploit the avenue of lobbying at various levels. The environmental implications of tourism development did not form part of the 1982 Policy.

The consequences are too obvious to be written about. However, the NAP, 1992 did carry specific provisions for environmental protection and harnessing. From Policy to Cartooning Policy statements may also lead to justifiable flights of fantasy. Two examples would illustrate how policies were used to justify stands taken by the politicians: a. Shri Devi Lal, the then Deputy Prime Minister wanted a 50% discount for farmers at Five Star Hotels run by India Tourism Development Corporation.

The scheme had teething problems since it was not easy to distinguish a farmer from amongst the clients who visit such hotels. However, on his insistence, the so-called CHAUPALs recreated a village ambience to the amazement of foreign tourists, who took a liking for them. b. Pursuing the objective of the Seventh Plan to diversify overseas tourism to its logical conclusion was what prompted A&. Jagdish Tytler to float the idea of casinos. It was an attempt to provide some entertainment for foreigners during the evenings. It was said that Indian classical music would not provide much needed entertainment for foreign guests because the artistes spend a lot of time tuning their instruments! Folk dances get over in an hour. So much for our much touted cultural diversity.

It is embarrassing to believe that the consultative committee attached to the Ministry of Civil Aviation and Tourism had endorsed the idea. Conclusion Broadly, our successive policy pronouncements in the realm of tourism falls within the "liberalising" framework of the macro-economic policy environment. The Finance Bill, 1988, had assured 50% tax exemption on foreign exchange earnings in the sector, and a further 50% exemption if re-invested. In effect, it amounts to 100% tax concession. Luxury hotels enjoy exemptions of all kinds with a view to encourage tourism earnings. These tax exemptions coupled with provision of soft loans to the sector led to a boom in the tourism related private investment. The Economic Survey 1991-92 aptly summarises the ultimate aim of such incentives for private sector participation: " The Government has tried to expand the economic space in which the people can exercise their initiative and ingenuity.

It hopes to do more to expand their opportunities, to enhance their potential. But what shape the economy takes ultimately depends on what the people make of it. In that sense, the future is in their hands." We should not forget that tourism is an industry which emerges in the context of unresolved socio-economic structural issues, such as land distribution patterns or the take over of traditional occupations by modem mechanised capital. Tourism happens to be a source of livelihood for millions in India and aggressive privatisation does not ensure social and economic safety nets. In the face of the unhindered entry of international capital and successive alienation, perhaps, it is difficult to agree that "the future is in our hands"

RURAL AREAS BENEFIT FROM RECREATION AND TOURISM DEVELOPMENT

Beautiful scenery-lakes, mountains, forests-attracts people to rural resort areas in the United States. Rural recreation areas have grown rapidly in recent years, and recreation and tourism development has become a popular vehicle for rural economic development.

Recreation development involves more than just tourist-related businesses, such as hotels and restaurants; it encompasses all economic growth that results from people moving into the community to take advantage of its recreational amenities. This kind of development has the potential to dramatically transform a stagnant rural community into a thriving community by attracting retirees, entrepreneurs, and young workers, diversifying the economy, and improving the quality of life with a broader array of goods and services.

But recreation development comes with potential problems. Some problems are growth-related-such as congested roads, crowded schools, environmental strains, housing shortages, despoiled scenic views, and conflicts over land use and public policies. Other problems are specific to the tourism industry's workers (unskilled or foreign), many of whom earn relatively little and have few fringe benefits. And another downside: Criminals may be particularly attracted to some recreation areas. Is recreation and tourism development a viable economic option for rural areas? ERS examined some key questions about the socioeconomic effects of rural recreation development. The answers are generally favourable, with improved employment conditions, earnings, and incomes; lower poverty rates; and healthier and better educated populations. However, conditions vary by type of recreation area, and higher housing costs and crime rates can accompany the more favourable outcomes.

DEFINITIONS AND METHODOLOGY

The word "recreation" is used in this article to refer to the leisure activities of tourists as well as seasonal and permanent residents. However, when discussing recreation's estimated impact on various socioeconomic indicators, the term 'recreation development' usually refers to the extent to which a county depends on recreation development for employment, income, and housing.

ERS used the 2002 version of its recreation county typology developed by Ken Johnson and Calvin Beale to analyze rural recreation areas nationwide. The number of recreation counties studied was 311, including 11 types varying by geographic location, natural amenities, and form of recreation.

ERS examined selected indicators of socioeconomic well-being in rural recreation areas nationwide, using county-level data from the 2000 Census and other Federal data sources. First, socioeconomic conditions and trends in rural recreation counties were compared with those in other nonmetro counties (excluding metro areas). Socioeconomic conditions and trends were also compared across various types of rural recreation counties. Next, multiple regression analysis was conducted to estimate the impact of recreation-dependency on socioeconomic conditions and trends in the 311 rural recreation counties. Because of rapid employment growth in rural recreation areas and a potentially broader array of jobs, including more seasonal and part-time positions that appeal to residents unable to work full-time, year-round jobs, employment options would likely be enhanced by recreation development. However, it may not be easier for residents to find jobs due to competition with other workers who have recently moved to the area. ERS researchers found that recreation development, measured by the extent to which a county's employment, income, and housing depend on recreation and tourism, is linked to a higher percentage of the working-age population having jobs. This percentage-employed measure encompasses discouraged workers who had dropped out of the labor force, making it a more comprehensive and meaningful measure of employment conditions. Moreover, recreation development led to an increase in this employment measure during the 1990s for all age groups, except the population ages 65 and older.

Jobs that are usually associated with recreation development, such as those in hotels and restaurants, are assumed to be low paying with few fringe benefits. Some related service jobs, such as those in retail businesses, may also pay low wages. However, low-wage workers in recreation areas may have access to more opportunities to work part-time and seasonal jobs to supplement their incomes, and some service and construction jobs associated with recreation development pay quite well. Recreation development appears to have increased the growth in earnings per job during the 1990s. But average earnings per job in 2000 were not significantly higher in rural recreation areas.

To better measure what residents earn from employment, ERS looked at total earnings per resident worker, which includes earnings from second jobs (part-time and seasonal). Second jobs are expected to be more readily available in recreation counties than elsewhere. Total earnings per resident were substantially higher ($2,000 more per worker) in recreation counties than in other rural counties. Contrary to conventional wisdom, recreation development seems to have increased residents' earnings.

COST OF LIVING HIGHER, BETTER EDUCATION AND HEALTH

Anecdotal evidence suggests that housing costs have risen rapidly in some of the most well-known recreation areas, becoming so high that many workers can no longer afford to live in the area, sometimes requiring long commutes. In addition, higher housing costs may prevent the children and grandchildren of some long-term residents from finding housing in their home towns. While this may be true in some recreation areas, it is not known how widespread this higher cost of living is. However, median rent for housing (an important component in cost of living) in recreation counties is 23 percent higher than in other nonmetropolitan (nonmetro) counties, reducing some of the economic advantages for recreation county residents, but only partially. Median household incomes are $3,185 higher in recreation counties than in other counties, while median annual rent is only $1,080 higher in recreation counties. This implies that the higher rent offsets about a third of the recreation county income advantage.

Recreational development might attract migrants who tend to have higher levels of education than nonmigrants. As expected, ERS research found that recreational development leads to a more educated population, particularly when education is measured by the share of adults with college degrees. Recreation development is also associated with good health (measured by age-adjusted death rates), as might be expected from the higher number of physicians (per 100,000 residents) in recreation counties than in other rural counties.

The availability of physicians, however, was not responsible for the good health of residents. Other factors, such as greater opportunities for physical exercise, may explain the health advantages associated with recreation development. In addition, the pristine environments of many recreation counties, with clean air and water, might lead to better overall health.

MORE CRIME, OTHER SOCIAL PROBLEMS

When recreation development is unplanned or occurs too rapidly, it can lead to congested roads and can strain the capacity of public services. Recreation areas have significantly higher rates of population growth than other rural areas, suggesting that some growth-related social problems, such as school crowding, housing shortages, pollution, and loss of identification with the community, may be present. ERS researchers examined road congestion by looking at commute times and found that recreation development was not linked to the commute time to work in 2000.

If anything, recreation development appears to have helped keep down commute times in recent years because recreation counties had smaller increases in average commute times during the 1990s than other rural counties. Recreation development can also result in higher poverty rates if significant numbers of low-wage, low-skilled workers arrive to work in tourist-related service establishments. However, ERS research indicates that recreation development results in significantly lower levels of poverty in rural recreation areas. In addition, recreation and tourism development appears to have contributed to declines in local poverty rates during the 1990s.

Another possible disadvantage is higher crime rates: Criminals may be drawn to recreation communities to prey on tourists, or certain types of recreation, such as casino gambling, could attract illicit activity. Crime rates (for serious crimes) are higher in recreation counties than in other rural counties. However, the way crime rates are calculated may be biased inherently against recreation areas. Crimes against tourists and seasonal residents are counted in the crime statistics, but tourists and seasonal residents are not counted as part of the population base upon which the crime rates are calculated.

Thus, even if people in recreation areas do not have a higher chance of becoming victims of crimes, the crime rates for these areas will appear higher than elsewhere because of this bias. Nevertheless, one could still argue that recreation-related crime adds to the local cost of policing and incarcerating criminals, just like recreation-related traffic adds to the cost of maintaining roads.

CONDITIONS VARY FROM PLACE TO PLACE

The benefits of recreation development for rural areas appear to be generally positive. This finding, along with the finding that socioeconomic effects vary significantly from one place to another, will inform policymakers seeking to achieve meaningful development through this strategy. The rural recreation counties in this analysis exhibit a considerable degree of diversity in socioeconomic conditions. For example, counties with ski resorts have among the wealthiest, best educated, and healthiest populations among all recreation county types. These counties also have relatively high crime rates.

In contrast, counties with reservoir-based recreation facilities (mainly located in parts of the Great Plains and the Midwest) and recreation counties in the southern Appalachian region have among the poorest, least educated residents among all recreation county types and relatively high age-adjusted death rates, but they have relatively low crime rates.

Counties with casino facilities had among the highest rates of job growth and large increases in earnings per job during the 1990s. Casino counties also had among the highest rates of growth in the share of employed people ages 65 and older, perhaps reflecting the greater need for jobs among older people in these high-poverty communities. Because recreation county types are not evenly distributed across the country, some of the differences may reflect interregional diversity.

This analysis focused on counties that have already succeeded in developing recreation as a significant industry. Most of these places have amenities that attract people. In contrast, some places that employ recreation as a development strategy may encounter difficulties because they lack natural amenities or other attributes that can attract large numbers of people. In these less attractive places, the socioeconomic benefits of recreation development are likely to be smaller.

9

Effects of Tourism on Economy

The tourism industry generates substantial economic benefits to both host countries and tourists' home countries. Especially in developing countries, one of the primary motivations for a region to promote itself as a tourism destination is the expected economic improvement.

As with other impacts, this massive economic development brings along both positive and negative consequences.

> *According to the World Tourism Organization, 698 million people traveled to a foreign country in 2000, spending more US$ 478 billion. International tourism receipts combined with passenger transport currently total more than US$ 575 billion-making tourism the world's number one export earner, ahead of automotive products, chemicals, petroleum and food.*
>
> ***Source:*** *WTTC*

NEGATIVE ECONOMIC IMPACTS OF TOURISM

There are many hidden costs to tourism, which can have unfavorable economic effects on the host community. Often rich countries are better able to profit from tourism than poor ones. Whereas the least developed countries have the most urgent need for income, employment and general rise of the standard of living by means of tourism, they are least able to realize these benefits. Among the reasons for this are large-scale transfer of tourism revenues out of the host country and exclusion of local businesses and products.

Leakage

The direct income for an area is the amount of tourist expenditure that remains locally after taxes, profits, and wages are paid outside the area and after imports are purchased; these subtracted amounts are called leakage. In most all-inclusive package tours, about 80% of travelers' expenditures go to the airlines, hotels and other international companies (who often have their headquarters in the travelers' home countries), and not to local businesses or workers. In addition, significant amounts of income actually retained at destination level can leave again through leakage.

A study of tourism 'leakage' in Thailand estimated that 70% of all money spent by tourists ended up leaving Thailand (via foreign-owned tour operators, airlines, hotels, imported drinks and food, etc.). Estimates for other Third World countries range from 80% in the Caribbean to 40% in India.

Source: *Sustainable Living*

Of each US$ 100 spent on a vacation tour by a tourist from a developed country, only around US$ 5 actually stays in a developing-country destination's economy. The figure below shows how the leakage happens.

There are two main ways that leakage occurs:

Import Leakage: This commonly occurs when tourists demand standards of equipment, food, and other products that the host country cannot supply. Especially in less-developed countries, food and drinks must often be imported, since local products are not up to the hotel's (i.e. tourist's) standards or the country simply doesn't have a supplying industry. Much of the income from tourism expenditures leaves the country again to pay for these imports.

The average import-related leakage for most developing countries today is between 40% and 50% of gross tourism earnings for small economies and between 10% and 20% for most advanced and diversified economies, according to UNCTAD.

> *Even in developed regions, local producers are often unable to supply the tourism industry appropriately even if good will is present: the 64-room hotel "Kaiser im Tirol" in Austria, an award-winning leader in sustainable practices, cannot find organic food suppliers in the local farming networks in the appropriate quantity, quality and reliability, as production cycles and processes are not compatible with its needs.*
>
> **Source:** *Austrian Preparatory Conference for the International Year of Ecotourism, September 2001*

Export leakage Multinational corporations and large foreign businesses have a substantial share in the import leakage. Often, especially in poor developing destinations, they are the only ones that possess the necessary capital to invest in the construction of tourism infrastructure and facilities. As a consequence of this, an export leakage arises when overseas investors who finance the resorts and hotels take their profits back to their country of origin.

> *A 1996 UN report evaluating the contribution of tourism to national income, gross levels of incomes or gross foreign exchange, found that net earnings of tourism, after deductions were made for all necessary foreign exchange expenditures, were much more significant for the industry. This report found significant leakage associated with: (a) imports of materials and equipment for construction; (b) imports of consumer goods, particularly food and drinks; (c) repatriation of profits earned by foreign investors; (d) overseas promotional expenditures and (e) amortization of external debt incurred in the development of hotels and resorts. The impact of the leakage varied greatly across countries, depending on the structure of the economy and the tourism*

industry. From the data presented in this study on the Caribbean, St. Lucia had a foreign exchange leakage rate of 56% from its gross tourism receipts, Aruba had 41%, Antigua and Barbuda 25% and Jamaica 40%.

Source: *Caribbean Voice*

Enclave Tourism: Local businesses often see their chances to earn income from tourists severely reduced by the creation of "all-inclusive" vacation packages. When tourists remain for their entire stay at the same cruise ship or resort, which provides everything they need and where they will make all their expenditures, not much opportunity is left for local people to profit from tourism.

The Organization of American States (OAS) carried out a survey of Jamaica's tourist industry that looked at the role of the all-inclusives compared to other types of accommodation. It found that 'All-inclusive hotels generate the largest amount of revenue but their impact on the economy is smaller per dollar of revenue than other accommodation subsectors.'

It also concluded that all-inclusives imported more, and employed fewer people per dollar of revenue than other hotels. This information confirms the concern of those who have argued that all-inclusives have a smaller trickle-down effect on local economies.

The cruise ship industry provides another example of economic enclave tourism. Non-river cruises carried some 8.7 million international passengers in 1999. On many ships, especially in the Caribbean (the world's most popular cruise destination with 44.5% of cruise passengers), guests are encouraged to spend most of their time and money on board, and opportunities to spend in some ports are closely managed and restricted.

OTHER NEGATIVE IMPACTS

Infrastructure Cost

Tourism development can cost the local government and local taxpayers a great deal of money. Developers may want the government to improve the airport, roads and other infrastructure, and possibly to provide tax breaks and other financial advantages, which are costly activities for the government. Public resources spent on subsidized infrastructure or tax breaks may reduce government investment in other critical areas such as education and health.

Increase in Prices

Increasing demand for basic services and goods from tourists will often cause price hikes that negatively affect local residents whose income does not increase proportionately. A San Francisco State University study of Belize found that, as a consequence of tourism development, the prices for locals increased by 8%.

Tourism development and the related rise in real estate demand may dramatically increase building costs and land values. Not only does this make it more difficult for local people, especially in developing countries, to meet their basic daily needs, it can also result in a dominance by outsiders in land markets and in-migration that erodes economic opportunities for the locals, eventually disempowering residents. In Costa Rica, close to 65% of the hotels belong to foreigners. Long-term tourists living in second homes, and the so-called amenity migrants (wealthy or retired people and liberal professionals moving to attractive destinations in order to enjoy the atmosphere and peaceful rhythms of life) cause price hikes in their new homes if their numbers attain a certain critical mass.

Economic Dependence of the Local Community

Diversification in an economy is a sign of health, however if a country or region becomes dependent for its economic survival upon one industry, it can put major stress upon this industry as well as the people involved to perform well. Many countries, especially developing countries with little ability to explore other resources, have embraced tourism as a way to boost the economy. In The Gambia, for instance, 30% of the workforce depends directly or indirectly on tourism.

In small island developing states, percentages can range from 83% in the Maldives to 21% in the Seychelles and 34% in Jamaica, according to the WTO. Over-reliance on tourism, especially mass tourism, carries significant risks to tourism-dependent economies. Economic recession and the impacts of natural disasters such as tropical storms and cyclones as well as changing tourism patterns can have a devastating effect on the local tourism sector.

Malta has only 380,000 residents, but received 1.2 million tourists in 1999. As 25% of GDP (and indirectly 40%), tourism generated more than $650 million in foreign exchange earnings. Malta's high dependence on tourism and a limited number of export products makes its trade performance vulnerable to shifts in international demand.

Source: *Washington Times*

Seasonal Character of Jobs

The seasonal character of the tourism industry creates economic problems for destinations that are heavily dependent on it. Problems that seasonal workers face include job (and therefore income) insecurity, usually with no guarantee of employment from one season to the next, difficulties in getting training, employment-related medical benefits, and recognition of their experience, and unsatisfactory housing and working conditions.

Other Industry Impacts Affecting Tourism

Economic crises, like the Asian crisis that hit Thailand, Malaysia and Indonesia a few years ago, can be devastating to inbound tourism flows. The financial turmoil triggered a sharp fall in tourism flows to affected countries during 1997 and 1998. In the Philippines, the crisis and the temporary closure of Philippine Airlines affected inbound arrivals significantly as there was a decline of almost 3.3% in 1998.

Source: *Hotel-online*

TOURISM CONTRIBUTION TO ECONOMIC CONSERVATION

The main positive economic impacts of tourism relate to foreign exchange earnings, contributions to government revenues, and generation of employment and business opportunities. These are discussed briefly here; further information on economic contributions from tourism can be found at the World Travel & Tourism Council's home page.

Foreign Exchange Earnings

Tourism expenditures and the export and import of related goods and services generate income to the host economy and can stimulate the investment necessary to finance growth in other economic sectors. Some countries seek to accelerate this growth by requiring visitors to bring in a certain amount of foreign currency for each day of their stay and do not allow them to take it out of the country again at the end of the trip.

> *An important indicator of the role of international tourism is its generation of foreign exchange earnings. Tourism is one of the top five export categories for as many as 83% of countries and is a main source of foreign exchange earnings for at least 38% of countries.*
>
> ***Source:** World Tourism Organization*

Contribution to Government Revenues

Government revenues from the tourism sector can be categorized as direct and indirect contributions. Direct contributions are generated by taxes on incomes from tourism employment and tourism businesses, and by direct levies on tourists such as departure taxes. Indirect contributions are those originated from taxes and duties levied on goods and services supplied to tourists.

The United States National Park Service estimates that the 273 million visits to American national parks in 1993 generated direct and indirect expenditures of US$ 10 billion and 200,000 jobs. When visits to land managed by other agencies, and to state, local, and privately-managed parks, are added, parks were estimated to bring around US$ 22 billion annually to the US economy. These expenditures also generate significant tax revenues for the government.

The World Travel and Tourism Council estimates that travel and tourism's direct, indirect, and personal tax contribution worldwide was over US$ 800 billion in 1998-a figure it expects to double by 2010. (Source: WTTC/Michigan State University Tax Policy Center)

Employment Generation

The rapid expansion of international tourism has led to significant employment creation. For example, the hotel accommodation sector alone provided around 11.3 million jobs worldwide in 1995. Tourism can generate jobs directly through hotels, restaurants, nightclubs, taxis, and souvenir sales, and indirectly through the supply of goods and services needed by tourism-related businesses. According to the WTO, tourism supports some 7% of the world's workers.

Stimulation of Infrastructure Investment

Tourism can induce the local government to make infrastructure improvements such as better water and sewage systems, roads, electricity, telephone and public transport networks, all of which can improve the quality of life for residents as well as facilitate tourism.

Contribution to Local Economies

Tourism can be a significant, even essential, part of the local economy. As the environment is a basic component of the tourism industry's assets, tourism revenues are often used to measure the economic value of protected areas. For example, Dorrigo National Park in New South Wales, Australia, has been estimated to contribute 7% of gross regional output and 8.4% of regional employment. The importance of tourism to local economies can also be illustrated by the impacts when it is disrupted: the catastrophic 1997 floods that closed Yosemite National Park in California cause locally severe economic losses to the areas around the park. In the most heavily impacted county, Mariposa County, 1997 personal income was reduced by an estimated US$1,159 per capita (US$18 million for the entire county)-a 6.6% decline. The county was also estimated to have lost US$1.67 million in county occupancy and sales tax revenues, and 956 jobs, a significant number in a county of fewer than 16,000 residents.

There are other local revenues that are not easily quantified, as not all tourist expenditures are formally registered in the macro-economic statistics. Money is earned from tourism through informal employment such as street vendors, informal guides, rickshaw drivers, etc. The positive side of informal or unreported employment is that the money is returned to the local economy, and has a great multiplier effect as it is spent over and over again. The World Travel and Tourism Council estimates that tourism generates an indirect contribution equal to 100% of direct tourism expenditures.

PURPOSES AND TYPES OF TOURISM

Adventure tourism is a type of niche tourism involving exploration or travel to remote areas, where the traveler should expect the unexpected. Adventure tourism is rapidly growing in popularity as tourists seek unusual holidays, different from the typical beach vacation.

Adventure tourism typically involves traveling into remote, inaccessible and possibly hostile areas. It may include the performance of acts that require significant effort and grit and may also involve some degree of risk.

According to the (U.S.-based) global Adventure Travel Trade Association, "adventure travel" may be any tourist activity including two of the following three components: a physical activity, a cultural exchange or interaction, and engagement with nature. Mountaineering expeditions, trekking, bungee jumping, rafting and rock climbing are frequently cited as an examples of adventure tourism.

MOUNTAINEERING

Mountaineering is the sport, hobby or profession of walking, hiking, trekking and climbing up mountains. It is also sometimes known as alpinism, particularly in Europe. It may be said to consist of three aspects: rock-craft, snow-craft and skiing, depending on whether the route chosen is over rock, snow or ice. All require great athletic and technical ability, and experience is also a very important part of the matter.

Technique

Snow

Snowshoes can be used to walk through deep snow approaching the mountain or on lesser slopes up the mountain. Skis can be used when conditions allow, and can be a form of the sport by itself, called Ski Mountaineering. Crampons can be used on hard snow (neve) and ice.

Glaciers

When traveling over glaciers, crevasses pose a grave danger. These giant cracks in the ice are not always visible as snow can be blown and freeze over the top to make a snowbridge. At times snowbridges can be as thin as a few inches.

Climbers use a system of ropes to protect themselves from such hazards. Basic gear for glacier travel includes crampons and ice axes. Teams of two to five climbers tie into a rope equally spaced. If a climber begins to fall the other members of the team perform a self-arrest to stop the fall. The other members of the team enact a crevasse rescue to pull the fallen climber from the crevasse.

Ice

Multiple methods are used to safely travel over ice. If the terrain is steep but not vertical protection in the form of pickets or ice screws can be driven into the snow or ice and attached to the rope by the lead climber. Each climber on the team must clip past the anchor, and the last climber picks up the picket.

This allows for safety should the entire team be taken off their feet. This technique is known as Simul-climbing. If the terrain becomes vertical then standard ice climbing techniques are used.

Shelter

Climbers use a few different forms of shelter depending on the situation and conditions. Shelter is a very important aspect of safety for the climber as the weather in the mountains is very unpredictable. Tall mountains require many days of camping on the mountain.

Hut

Particularly the European alpine regions have a tight network of mountain huts, in most cases managed by full time, seasonal employees. These huts offer shelter, warm and cold meals, rooms or sleeping dormitories and sanitary facilities. In terms of luxury and comfort they vary by a great deal. Most huts are only open during the spring, summer and fall months to serve recreational mountaineers but also offer a self-service section to provide shelter and a cooking place for winter mountaineers. Using the hut system enables the mountaineer to travel without heavy tent, sleeping bag and cooking supplies.

Bivy

A bivy or bivouac is simply getting a sleeping bag and Bivouac sack and laying down to sleep. Many times small half sheltered areas like cracks in rocks or simply a trench dug in the snow are used to provide a basic means of shelter as well. This technique is performed by most people only in cases of emergency, however in good weather this can be pleasant. Some climbers steadfastly committed to Alpine Style climbing plan on bivying in order to save the weight of a tent when snow conditions are not suitable for a snow cave.

Tent

Tents are the most common form of shelter used on the mountain. A four season tent is required for any camp high in the mountains. Many climbers do not use tents at high altitudes unless the snow conditions do not allow for snow caving. One of the downsides to tenting is that storm winds can be very unnerving and can cause the tent to collapse, however modern mountaineering tents are usually tested for wind speeds up to 125mph. Even so, very intense flapping of the tent fabric can hinder sleep and raise doubts about the security of the shelter in windy conditions.

Snow cave

Snow caves are the preferred way for many climbers to shelter high on the mountain. Unlike tents snow caves are silent and are actually much warmer than a tent. A correctly made snow cave will hover around freezing, which relative to outside temperatures can be very warm. Igloos are used by some climbers, but are deceptively difficult to build and require specific snow conditions.

Hazards

The craft of climbing has been developed to avoid three main types of danger: the danger of things falling on the climber (objective danger), the danger of the climber falling and inclement weather. The things that may fall include rocks, ice, snow, other climbers or their gear; the mountaineer may fall from rocks, ice or snow, or into a crevasse. In all, there are eight chief dangers: falling rocks, falling ice, snow-avalanches, falls,the climber falling, falls from ice slopes, falls down snow slopes, falls into crevasses and dangers from weather. To select and follow a route using one's skills and experience to mitigate these dangers is to exercise the climber's craft.

Falling Rocks

Every rock mountain is slowly disintegrating due to erosion, the process being especially rapid above the snow-line. Rock faces are constantly swept by falling stones, which are generally possible to dodge. Falling rocks tend to form furrows in a mountain face, and these furrows (couloirs) have to be ascended with caution, their sides often being safe when the middle is stoneswept. Rocks fall more frequently on some days than on others, according to the recent weather. Ice formed during the night may temporarily bind rocks to the face but warmth of the day or direct sun exposure may easily dislodge these rocks. Local experience is a valuable help on determining typical rockfall on such routes.

The direction of the dip of rock strata often determines the degree of danger on a particular face; the character of the rock must also be considered. Where stones fall frequently debris will be found below, whilst on snow slopes falling stones cut furrows visible from a great distance. In planning an ascent of a new peak mountaineers must look for such traces. When falling stones get mixed in considerable quantity with slushy snow or water a mud avalanche is formed (common in the Himalaya). It is vital to avoid camping in their possible line of fall.

Falling Ice

The places where ice may fall can always be determined beforehand. It falls in the broken parts of glaciers (seracs) and from overhanging cornices formed on the crests of narrow ridges. Large icicles are often formed on steep rock faces, and these fall frequently in fine weather following cold and stormy days. They have to be avoided like falling stones. Seracs are slow in formation, and slow in arriving (by glacier motion) at a condition of unstable equilibrium.

They generally fall in or just after the hottest part of the day, and their debris seldom goes far. A skillful and experienced ice-man will usually devise a safe route through a most intricate ice-fall, but such places should be avoided in the afternoon of a hot day. Hanging glaciers (i.e. glaciers perched on steep slopes) often discharge themselves over steep rock-faces, the snout breaking off at intervals. They can always be detected by their debris below. Their track should be avoided.

Avalanches

The avalanche is the most underestimated danger in the mountains. People generally think that they will be able to recognize the hazards and survive being caught. The truth is a somewhat different story. Every year, 120-150 people die in small avalanches in the Alps alone. The vast majority are reasonably experienced male skiers aged 20-35 but also include ski instructors and guides. There is always a lot of pressure to risk a snow crossing. Turning back takes a lot of extra time and effort, supreme leadership, and most importantly there seldom is an avalanche to prove the right decision was made. Making the decision to turn around is especially hard if others are crossing the slope, but any next person could become the trigger.

There are two types of avalanche:

1. *The Slab Avalanche:* This type of avalanche occurs when a plate of snow breaks loose and starts sliding down; these are the largest and most dangerous.
    1. Hard Slab Avalanche-formed by hard-packed snow in a cohesive slab. The slab will not break up easily as it slides down the hill, resulting in large blocks tumbling down the mountain.
    2. Soft Slab Avalanche-formed again by a cohesive layer of snow bonded together, the slab tends to break up more easily.
2. *The Loose Snow Avalanche:* This type of avalanche is triggered by a small amount of moving snow that accumulates into a big slide. Also known as a "wet slide or point release" avalanche. This type of avalanche is deceptively dangerous as it can still knock a climber or skier off their feet and bury them, or sweep them over a cliff into a terrain trap.

Dangerous slides are most likely to occur on the same slopes preferred by many skiers: long and wide open, few trees or large rocks, 30 to 45 degrees of angle, large load of fresh snow, soon after a big storm, on a slope 'lee to the storm'. Solar radiation can trigger slides as well.

These will typically be a point release or wet slough type of avalanche. The added weight of the wet slide can trigger a slab avalanche. Ninety percent of reported victims are caught in avalanches triggered by themselves or others in their group.

When going off-piste or traveling in alpine terrain, parties have a moral responsibility to always carry:

1. avalanche beacon
2. probe

3. shovel (retrieving victims with a shovel instead of your hands is five times faster)

and to have had avalanche training! Paradoxically, expert skiers who have avalanche training make up a large percentage of avalanche fatalities; perhaps because they are the ones more likely to ski in areas prone to avalanches.

Even with proper rescue equipment and training, there is a one-in-five chance of dying if caught in a significant avalanche, and only a 50/50 chance of being found alive if buried more than a few minutes. The best solution is to learn how to avoid risky conditions.

Falls from Rocks

The skill of a rock climber is shown by one's choice of handhold and foothold, and his adhesion to those one has chosen. Much depends on a correct estimate of the firmness of the rock where weight is to be thrown upon it.

Many loose rocks are quite firm enough to bear a person's weight, but experience is needed to know which can be trusted, and skill is required in transferring the weight to them without jerking. On rotten rocks the rope must be handled with special care, lest it should start loose stones on to the heads of those below. Similar care must be given to handholds and footholds, for the same reason.

When a horizontal traverse has to be made across very difficult rocks, a dangerous situation may arise unless at both ends of the traverse there be firm positions. Mutual assistance on hard rocks takes all manner of forms: two, or even three, people climbing on one another's shoulders, or using an ice axe propped up by others for a foothold.

The great principle is that of co-operation, all the members of the party climbing with reference to the others, and not as independent units; each when moving must know what the climber in front and the one behind are doing. After bad weather steep rocks are often found covered with a veneer of ice (verglas), which may even render them inaccessible. Crampons are useful on such occasions.

Ice Slopes

For travel on slopes consisting of ice or hard snow, crampons are a standard part of a mountaineer's equipment. While step-cutting can sometimes be used on snow slopes of moderate angle, this can be a slow and tiring process, which does not provide the higher security of crampons. However, in soft snow or powder, crampons are easily hampered by balling of snow which reduce their effectiveness. In either case, an ice axe not only assists with balance but provides the climber with the possibility of self-arrest in case of a slip or fall. On a true ice slope however, an ice axe is rarely able to effect a self-arrest. As an additional safety precaution on steep ice slopes, the climbing rope is attached to ice screws buried into the ice.

True ice slopes are rare in Europe, though common in mountains located in the tropics, where newly-fallen snow quickly thaws on the surface and becomes sodden below, so that the next night's frost turns the whole mass into a sheet of semi-solid ice.

Snow Slopes

Snow slopes are very common, and usually easy to ascend. At the foot of a snow or ice slope is generally a big crevasse, called a bergschrund, where the final slope of the mountain rises from a snow-field or glacier. Such bergschrunds are generally too wide to be stepped across, and must be crossed by a snow bridge, which needs careful testing and a painstaking use of the rope. A steep snow slope in bad condition may be dangerous, as the whole body of snow may start as an avalanche. Such slopes are less dangerous if ascended directly than obliquely, for an oblique or horizontal track cuts them across and facilitates movement of the mass.

New snow lying on ice is especially dangerous. Experience is needed for deciding on the advisability of advancing over snow in doubtful condition. Snow on rocks is usually rotten unless it is thick; snow on snow is likely to be sound. A day or two of fine weather will usually bring new snow into sound condition. Snow cannot lie at a very steep angle, though it often deceives the eye as to its slope. Snow slopes seldom exceed 40°. Ice slopes may be much steeper. Snow slopes in early morning are usually hard and safe, but the same in the afternoon are quite soft and possibly dangerous; hence the advantage of an early start.

Crevasses

Crevasses are the slits or deep chasms formed in the substance of a glacier as it passes over an uneven bed. They may be open or hidden. In the lower part of a glacier the crevasses are open. Above the snow-line they are frequently hidden by arched-over accumulations of winter snow. The detection of hidden crevasses requires care and experience.

After a fresh fall of snow they can only be detected by sounding with the pole of the ice axe, or by looking to right and left where the open extension of a partially hidden crevasse may be obvious. The safeguard against accident is the rope, and no one should ever cross a snow-covered glacier unless roped to one, or even better to two companions. Anyone venturing onto crevasses should be trained in crevasse rescue.

Weather

The primary dangers caused by bad weather centre around the changes it causes in snow and rock conditions, making movement suddenly much more arduous and hazardous than under normal circumstances.

Whiteouts make it difficult to retrace a route while rain may prevent taking the easiest line only determined as such under dry conditions. In a storm the mountaineer who uses a compass for guidance has a great advantage over a merely empirical observer. In large snow-fields it is, of course, easier to go wrong than on rocks, but intelligence and experience are the best guides in safely navigating objective hazards.

Summer thunderstorms may produce intense lightning. If a climber happens to be standing on or near the summit, they risk being struck.

There are many cases where people have been struck by lightning while climbing mountains. In most mountainous regions, local storms develop by late morning and early afternoon. Many climbers will get an "alpine start"; that is before or by first light so as to be on the way down when storms are intensifying in activity and lightning and other weather hazards are a distinct threat to safety.

Altitude

Rapid ascent can lead to altitude sickness. The best treatment is to descend immediately. The climber's motto at high altitude is "climb high, sleep low", referring to the regimen of climbing higher to acclimatize but returning to lower elevation to sleep. In the South American Andes, the chewing of coca leaves has been traditionally used to treat altitude sickness symptoms. Common symptoms of altitude sickness include severe headache, sleep problems, nausea, lack of appetite, lethargy and body ache. Mountain sickness may progress to HACE (High Altitude Cerebral Edema) and HAPE (High Altitude Pulmonary Edema), both of which can be fatal within 24 hours. In high mountains, atmospheric pressure is lower and this means that less oxygen is available to breathe. This is the underlying cause of altitude sickness. Everyone needs to acclimatize, even exceptional mountaineers that have been to high altitude before. Generally speaking, mountaineers start using bottled oxygen when they climb above 7,000 m. Exceptional mountaineers have climbed 8000-metre peaks (including Everest) without oxygen, almost always with a carefully planned program of acclimatization. In 2005, researcher and mountaineer John Semple established that above-average ozone concentrations on the Tibetan plateau may pose an additional risk to climbers.

Locations

Mountaineering has become a popular sport throughout the world. In Europe the sport largely originated in the Alps, and is still immensely popular there. Other notable mountain ranges frequented by climbers include the Caucasus, the Pyrenees and the Tatra mountains. In North America climbers frequent the Rockies and Sierra Nevada of California, the Cascades of Washington and the high peaks of Alaska. There has been a long tradition of climbers going on expeditions to the Greater Ranges, a term generally used for the Andes and the high peaks of Asia including the Himalaya, Pamirs and Tien Shan. In the past this was often on exploratory trips or to make first ascents. With the advent of cheaper long-haul air travel mountaineering holidays in the Greater Ranges are now undertaken much more frequently and ascents of even Everest and Vinson Massif (the highest mountain in Antarctica) are offered as a "package holiday". Other popular mountaineering areas of more local interest include the Southern Alps of New Zealand, the Japanese Alps the Scottish Highlands and the mountains of Scandinavia.

History

- Though it is unknown whether his intention was to reach a summit, Ötzi ascended at least 3,000 m in the Alps about 5,300 years ago. His remains were found at that altitude, preserved in a glacier.
- The first recorded mountain ascent in the Common Era is Roman Emperor Hadrian's ascent of Etna (3,350 m) to see the sun rise in 121.
- Peter III of Aragon climbed Canigou in the Pyrenees in the last quarter of the 13th century.
- The first ascent of the Popocatépetl (5,426 m in Mexico) was reported in 1289 by members of a local tribe (Tecanuapas)
- Jean Buridan climbed Mont Ventoux around 1316.
- The Italian poet Petrarch wrote that on April 26, 1336 he, together with his brother and two servants, climbed to the top of Mont Ventoux (1,909 m). His account of the trip was composed later as a letter to his friend Francesco Dionigi. Subsequently, April 26, 1336 came to be regarded as the "birth of alpinism", and Petrarch (Petrarca alpinista) as the "father of alpinism".
- The Rochemelon (3,538 m) in the Italian Alps was climbed in 1358.
- In the late 1400s and early 1500s ascents were made of numerous high peaks in the Andes, for religious

purposes by the citizens of the Inca Empire and their subjects. They constructed platforms, houses and altars on many summits and carried out sacrifices, including human sacrifices. The highest peak they are known for certain to have climbed is Llullaillaco (6,739 m). They may also have ascended the highest peak in the Andes, Aconcagua (6,962 m) as a sacrifice victim has been found at over 5,000 m on this peak.

- In 1492 the ascent of Mont Aiguille was made by order of Charles VIII of France. The Humanists of the 16th century adopted a new attitude towards mountains, but the disturbed state of Europe nipped in the bud the nascent mountaineering of the Zurich school.
- Leonardo da Vinci climbed to a snow-field in the neighborhood of the Val Sesia and made scientific observations.
- In 1642 Darby Field made the first recorded ascent of Mount Washington, then known as Agiocochook, in New Hampshire.
- Konrad Gesner and Josias Simler of Zurich visited and described mountains, and made regular ascents. The use of ice axe and rope were locally invented at this time. No mountain expeditions of note are recorded in the 17th century.
- Richard Pococke and William Windham's historic visit to Chamonix was made in 1741, and set the trend for visiting glaciers.
- In 1744 the Titus was climbed, the first true ascent of a snow-mountain.
- The first attempt to ascend Mont Blanc was made in 1775 by a party of natives. In 1786 Dr Michel Paccard and Jacques Balmat gained the summit for the first time. Horace-Bénédict de Saussure, the initiator of the first ascent followed next year.
- The Norwegian mountain climber, Jens Esmark was the first person to ascend Snøhetta in 1798, part of the Dovrefjell range in Southern Norway. The same year

he lead the first expedition to Bitihorn, a small mountain in the southernmost outskirts of Jotunheimen, Norway. In 1810 he was the first person to ascend Mount Gaustatoppen in Telemark, Norway.

- The Jungfrau was climbed in 1811, the Finsteraarhorn in 1812, and the Breithorn in 1813. Thereafter, tourists showed a tendency to climb, and the body of Alpine guides began to come into existence as a consequence.
- Citlaltépetl (5720 m in Mexico) was first climbed in 1848 by F. Maynard & G. Reynolds.
- Systematic mountaineering, as a sport, is usually dated from Sir Alfred Wills's ascent of the Wetterhorn in 1854. The first ascent of Monte Rosa was made in 1855.
- The Alpine Club was founded in London in 1857, and was soon imitated in most European countries. Edward Whymper's ascent of the Matterhorn in 1865 marked the close of the main period of Alpine conquest-the Golden age of alpinism-during which the craft of climbing was invented and 'perfected', the body of professional guides formed and their traditions fixed.
- Passing to other ranges, the exploration of the Pyrenees was concurrent with that of the Alps. The Caucasus followed, mainly owing to the initiative of D. W. Freshfield; it was first visited by exploring climbers in 1868, and most of its great peaks were climbed by 1888.
- The Edelweiss Club Salzburg was founded in Salzburg in 1881, and had 3 members make the First Ascent on 2 Eight-thousanders, Broad Peak (1957) and Dhaulagiri (1960).
- Trained climbers turned their attention to the mountains of North America in 1888, when the Rev. W. S. Green made an expedition to the Selkirk Mountains. From that time exploration has gone on apace, and many English and American climbing parties have surveyed most of the highest peaks; Pikes Peak (14,115 ft.) having been climbed by Mr. E. James and party in 1820, and Mt. Saint Elias (18,008 ft.) by the Duke of the Abruzzi

and party in 1897. The exploration of the highest Andes was begun in 1879-1880, when Whymper climbed Chimborazo and explored the mountains of Ecuador. The Cordillera between Chile and Argentina was visited by Dr. Gussfeldt in 1883, who ascended Maipo (17,270 ft.) and attempted Aconcagua (22,841 ft.). That peak was first climbed by the Fitzgerald expedition in 1897.

- The Andes of Bolivia were first explored by Sir William Martin Conway in 1898. Chilean and Argentine expeditions revealed the structure of the southern Cordillera in the years 1885-1898. Conway visited the mountains of Tierra del Fuego.
- New Zealand's Southern Alps were first visited in 1882 by the Rev. W. S. Green, and shortly afterwards a New Zealand Alpine Club was founded, and by their activities the exploration of the range was pushed forward. In 1895, Major Edward Arthur Fitzgerald, made an important journey in this range. Tom Fyfe and party climbed Aoraki/Mount Cook on Christmas Day 1894, denying Fitzgerald the first ascent. Fitzgerald was en route from Britain with Swiss guide Matthias Zurbriggen to claim the peak. So piqued at being beaten to the top of Mount Cook, he refused to climb it and concentrated on other peaks in the area. Later in the trip Zubriggen soloed Mount Cook up a ridge that now bears his name.
- The first mountains of the arctic region explored were those of Spitzbergen by Sir W. M. Conway's expeditions in 1896 and 1897.
- Of the high African peaks, Kilimanjaro was climbed in 1889 by Dr. Hans Meyer, Mt. Kenya in 1899 by Halford John Mackinder, and a peak of Ruwenzori by H. J. Moore in 1900.
- The Asiatic mountains were initially surveyed on orders of the British Empire. In 1892 Sir William Martin Conway explored the Karakoram Himalaya, and climbed a peak of 23,000 ft. In 1895 Albert F. Mummery died while attempting Nanga Parbat, while in 1899 D. W.

Freshfield took an expedition to the snowy regions of Sikkim. In 1899, 1903, 1906 and 1908 Mrs Fannie Bullock Workman made ascents in the Himalayas, including one of the Nun Kun peaks (23,300 ft.). A number of Gurkha sepoys were trained as expert mountaineers by Major the Hon. C. G. Bruce, and a good deal of exploration was accomplished by them.

- The Rucksack Club was founded in Manchester, England in 1902.
- The American Alpine Club was founded in 1902.
- In 1902, the Eckenstein-Crowley Expedition, lead by mountaineer Oscar Eckenstein and occultist Aleister Crowley, was the first to attempt to scale Chogo Ri (now known as K2 in the west). They reached 22,000 feet before turning back due to weather and other mishaps.
- In 1905, Aleister Crowley led the first expedition to Kanchenjunga, the third highest mountain in the world. Four members of that party were killed in an avalanche. Some claims say they reached around 21,300 feet before turning back, however Crowley's autobiography claims they reached about 25,000 feet.
- The 1950s saw the first ascents of all the eight-thousanders but two, starting with Annapurna in 1950 by Maurice Herzog and Louis Lachenal. The world's highest mountain (above mean sea level), Mount Everest (8,848 m) was first climbed on May 29, 1953 by Sir Edmund Hillary and Tenzing Norgay from the south side in Nepal. Just a few months later, Hermann Buhl made the first ascent of Nanga Parbat (8,125 m), a remarkable solo climb, the only eight-thousander to be solo'd on the first ascent. K2 (8,611 m), the second highest peak in the world was first scaled in 1954. In 1964, the final eight-thousander to be climbed was Shishapangma (8,013 m), the lowest of all the 8,000 metre peaks.

10

Tourism and its Rapid Growth

AGRITOURISM

Agritourism is a style of vacation in which hospitality is offered on farms. This may include the opportunity to assist with farming tasks during the visit. Agritourism is often practiced in wine growing regions, as in Italy, France and Spain. In America, Agritourism is wide-spread and includes any farm open to the public at least part of the year.

Tourists can pick fruits and vegetables, ride horses, taste honey, learn about wine, shop in gift shops and farm stands for local and regional produce or hand-crafted gifts, and much more. Agritourism is being developed as a valuable component of a business model to support many agricultural entities when the farm products they produce are no longer economically competitive otherwise. To help promote the single agritourism operations, some farms get together to form festivals, tours or other events.

People are more interested in how their food is produced and want to meet the producers and talk with them about what goes into food production. Children who visit the farms often have not seen a live duck, or goat, and have not picked an apple right off the tree. This form of expanded agri-tourism has given birth to what are often called "entertainment farms." These farms cater to the pick-your-own crowd, offering not only regular farm products, but also food, mazes, open-pen animals, train rides, picnic facilities and pick-your-own produce. Dude ranches offer tourists the chance to work on cattle ranches and sometimes include cattle drives.

ARCHAEOLOGICAL TOURISM

Archaeotourism or Archaeological tourism is an alternative form of cultural tourism, which aims to promote the passion for historical-archaeology and the conservation of historical sites.

Establishment

Investigator Georgeos Diaz-Montexano, who initiated a series of publications in 1995 about ArchaeoTourism, such as "Arqueología y Enigmas de la Historia", "Arqueología Sin Fronteras", "La Esfinge. Revista de Egiptologia" and "ArqueoHistoria", brought awareness to the concept of archaeological tourism. Shortly after writing these publications, he founded the first specialized society on Archaeotourism, ArqueoTour (2000). For these efforts, he is considered by some to be the founder of archaeotourism.

Like Ecological tourism (or Ecotourism), Archaeological tourism is promoted to encourage the development of cultural associations, and companies and cooperatives can be found that dedicate themselves to offer this type of service.

The best definition of archaeotourism can be found in the words of its founders:

The passion by the past is something inherent to the human being. As it says well: "Town that does not know from where town comes that does not know to where it goes".

The Archaeotourism or archaeological tourism is ideal for which they look for a higher knowledge and sublimates, tie to the meditation and the relaxation, in perfect syntony with the surroundings or ecosystem that is, integration with the Mother Nature, but always in old places, next to the ruins of the "enigmatic missing civilizations".

Sites and places magician-monks or asylums. From the most remote prehistoric times. From the era of the dinosaurios to the Medieval Age. In order to develop his activities it has a nourished group of authentic experts in each one of the matters.

Therefore, archaeologists, paleontologists, anthropologists, historians and specialists in trips will unite their knowledge under a same objective: to offer to the traveller a wonderful and unforgettable experience, an intensive course and of introduction to each one of these manifestations of the human knowledge. This way the visitor will not be a simple traveller, will be in addition an apprentice in sciences to the past.

Some times will feel a paleontologist discovering tracks of dinosaurious and others will feel like Indiana Jones in the Damn Temple, mainly when penetrating in the mysterious caverns and artificial caves that long ago served from temples our ancestors. Enigmatic places loaded of an atmosphere of magic and mystery that, sometimes, surpass to all fiction created by the cinema...

Other Definitions

Archaeological tourism can include all products associated with public archaeological promotion, including visits to archaeological sites, museums, interpretation centers, reinactment of historical occurrences, the rediscovery of native products, festivals, or theater.

Although archaeological tourism is quite recent, many international institutions and governments have already begun to contemplate viable alternative activity for the sustainable economic-social development. Several countries have for years had programs resembling the main points of Archaeological tourism for economic income, including Egypt, Mexico and Peru.

BOOKSTORE TOURISM

Bookstore tourism is a type of cultural tourism that promotes independent bookstores as a group travel destination. It started as a grassroots effort to support locally owned and operated bookshops, many of which have struggled to compete with large bookstore chains and online retailers.

The project was initiated in 2003 by Larry Portzline, a writer and college instructor in Harrisburg, Pennsylvania who led "bookstore road trips" to other cities and recognized its potential as a group travel niche and marketing tool. He promoted the concept with a how-to book and a web site, and groups around the U.S. soon began offering similar excursions, usually via a chartered bus, and often incorporating book signings, author home tours, and historical sites. In 2005-06, the Southern California Booksellers Association and Northern California Independent Booksellers Association embraced bookstore tourism, offering trips to independent bookstores in Los Angeles, San Diego and San Francisco.

The Bookstore Tourism movement encourages schools, libraries, reading groups, and organizations of all sizes to create day-trips and literary outings to cities and towns with a concentration of independent bookstores. It also encourages local booksellers to attract bibliophiles to their communities by employing bookstore tourism as an economic development tool. Others benefiting include local retailers, restaurants, bus companies, and travel professionals.

The effort also provides organizations with an outreach opportunity to support reading and literacy. Portzline has traveled across the country to promote the concept. In Fall 2006 he launched the National Council on Bookstore Tourism (NCBT), a nonprofit organization and trade association that will partner with booksellers, libraries, educators, literary festivals, the travel industry and economic development agencies at the national, state and local levels. In 2006 he created a promotional video featuring group "bookstore road trips" in New York City's Greenwich Village and in Los Angeles area "beach towns" and posted it on the NCBT website.

CULTURAL TOURISM

'Cultural tourism' (or culture tourism) is the subset of tourism concerned with a country or region's culture, especially its arts. It generally focuses on traditional communities who has diverse customs, unique form of art and distinct social practices, which basically distinguishes it from other types/

forms of culture. Cultural tourism includes tourism in urban areas, particularly historic or large cities and their cultural facilities such as museums and theatres. It can also include tourism in rural areas showcasing the traditions of indigenous cultural communities (i.e. festivals, rituals), and their values and lifestyle. It is generally agreed that cultural tourists spend substantially more than standard tourists do. This form of tourism is also becoming generally more popular throughout Europe.

Destination

Definition

By definition, the term destination refers broadly to any given area where tourism is a relatively important activity, like for instance having an economy significantly influenced by tourism revenues. However, it is complicated by the fact that a single, recognizable destination may include several cities, towns or municipalities, provinces, or other government entities-in island archipelago it may be the entire country.

Types

Living Cultural Areas

Due to globalization, technology and the onset of cultural tourism and ecotourism, the number of living cultural areas is continually declining. For an indigenous culture that has stayed largely separated from the surrounding majority, tourism can present both advantages and problems. On the positive side are the unique cultural practices and arts that attract the curiosity of tourists and provide opportunities for tourism and economic development. On the negative side is the issue of how to control tourism so that those same cultural amenities are not destroyed and the people do not feel violated.

Prominent Examples

Chiloé, Chile

Chiloé is Chile's largest island, located at the midway point between the capital, Santiago, and the country's extreme south at Tierra del Fuego. Chiloé is the site of the Chiloé Model

Forest, member of the same network as the Calakmul and Eastern Ontario Model Forests. Having evolved for centuries isolated from mainland Chile, the "Chilotes" developed a strong, self-reliant culture, rich in folklore, mythology and tradition. This very identity is what constitutes the island's major attraction for domestic tourists in Chile and increasingly, for international tourists.

As in the Calakmul case above, tourism to Chiloé is very strongly based on the island's cultural heritage, predominantly consisting of crafts markets, appreciation of cultural landscapes, museum exhibitions, seafood cuisine and architectural heritage (Chiloé's old churches). However, the average tourist to the island will have little opportunity to see Chilotes involved in their living cultural activities, such as the elaborate preparation of the islands famous "curanto" meal, rich in shellfish, meat and potatoes, the management practices of their farm and forest lands, boat building and more.

In order to overcome the cultural and organizational barriers that keep suppliers of living cultural heritage and tour operators apart, the Chiloé diocese of Ancud established a private foundation called "Fundación con Todos" (One for All Foundation). Among other activities, the Foundation has played a key role in helping a number of Chilote households organize themselves into an "agrotourism" network. The Foundation helped Chilote households make the preparation required to accommodate tourists (including training in sanitation and maintenance of facilities, the provision of basic infrastructure) and complemented this effort with a professional marketing campaign. These works were undertaken with the financial support of other agencies.

Again, in cooperation with the EOMF and the Chiloé Model Forest, a cultural and natural heritage tour was organized to Argentina and Chile, including a three-day visit to Chiloé, permitting some of the Chilote households to host a group of cultural heritage tourists for the first time. The visits were very successful and should be the first of more to come, helping establish the credibility of Chiloé's agrotourism network among other tour operators.

Orrissa Tribes

Nestling on the eastern coast of India, Orissa is one of the most exquisite regions dominated by exotic sandy beaches, plenteous wild life, and holy temples famous for their architectural splendor and primitive lifestyle. The charm of the city is still well-nigh chaste and unrevealed by the visitors, up to its full extent.

The other lure of the city lies in its tribal population dotted with more than 62 tribal communities. The tribal communities of Orissa constitute about 23% of its total population. Orissa is inhabited by tribes like Saora or Sabar that had a respectable mentioning in the epic of Mahabharata.

Mostly the Orissa tribes are high land habitats with opulent ethnic trait, cultures and customs dominated by varying languages. The culture conscious tribes are able to preserve their social customs and dignified values. The most primitive tribes are Bondas, Gadabas, Koyas, Kondhas and Sauras.

The culture of tribal Orissa is affluent with their own folk songs and dances, their tattoos. Tribal culture of Orissa is well depicted in its modern city in form of poems, art and craft or music. The tribes have adapted the Hindu traditions and culture from centuries, which is mixed with their own culture giving a distinct zest to the entire racial. Songs and dances are the essence of the tribal culture of Orissa. The traditions and the ceremonies for wedding, birth and death all are represented by singing songs, rural dances along with feasts.

The Tribal Folk Orissan tribes are strong, assiduous and simple hospitable tribes, normally like to be reserved and maintain distance from the people of other communities, as they are too shy.

The major occupation of these tribes is agriculture and fishing and hunting. Men usually wear loin attire and women rap long stretch of cloth around them. Women are adorned with ornaments like bangles, armlets, bracelets, necklaces, rings, hairpins etc usually made of silvers, aluminum, and brass. The practice of tattooing is prevalent among women folk. Girls above 5 years are found with tattoo mark on their faces and hands. Festival Celebration Numbers of deities are worshiped by the tribes for their happy life. Many festivals are also celebrated with much of enthusiasm and excitement. The ceremony rituals are observed through out the year in order to appease their deities and ascendant.

The most significant festival of the year are the chaita parab and push parab-this day all able men of the village go on a hunting expedition. The tribes with their cultural dance, song and music all distinguish custom of their artistic life, which demarcate them from the other non tribal groups. Orissa acquire every thing Orissa is a state, embellished with hilly terrain of the Eastern Ghats, where primitive tribes dwell and a beautiful stretch of the Indo-Aryans coast where modern life persists. A blend of 2 discrete civilization with contrast cultures, beautiful landscapes, beaches, rich wildlife, offers the best of India to its visitors.

Destination Planning

As the issue of globalization takes place to this modern time, the challenge of preserving the few remaining cultural community around the world is becoming hard. In a tribal based community, reaching economic advancement with minimal negative impacts is an essential objective to any destination planner.

Since they are using the culture of the region as the main attraction, sustainable destination development of the area is vital for them to prevent the negative impacts (i.e. destroying the authentic identity of the tribal community) due to tourism.

Management Issues

Certainly, the principle of "one size fits all" doesn't apply to destination planning. The needs, expectations, and anticipated benefits from tourism vary greatly from one destination to another. This is clearly exemplified as local communities living in regions with tourism potential (destinations) develop a vision for what kind of tourism they want to facilitate, depending on issues and concerns they want to be settled or satisfied.

Destination Planning Resources

Planning Guides

It is important that the destination planner takes into account the diverse definition of culture as the term is subjective. Satisfying tourists' interests such as landscapes, seascapes, art, nature, traditions, ways of life and other products associated to them-which may be categorized cultural in the broadest sense of the word, is a prime consideration as it marks the initial phase of the development of a cultural destination.

The quality of service and destination, which doesn't solely depend on the cultural heritage but more importantly to the cultural environment, can further be developed by setting controls and policies which shall govern the community and its stakeholders. It is therefore safe to say that the planner should be on the ball with the varying meaning of culture itself as this fuels the formulation of development policies that shall entail efficient planning and monitored growth (e.g. strict policy on the protection and preservation of the community).

Local community, tourists, the destination and sustainable tourism.

While satisfying tourists' interests and demands may be a top priority, it is also imperative to ruminate the subsystems of the destination's (residents). Development pressures should be anticipated and set to their minimum level so as to conserve the area's resources and prevent a saturation of the destination as to not abuse the product and the residents correspondingly. The plan should incorporate the locals to its gain by training and employing them and in the process encourage them to participate to the travel business. Keep in mind that the plan should make travellers not only aware about the destination but also concern on how to help it sustain its character while broadening their travelling experience.

Planning Tools

The core of a planner's job is to design an appropriate planning process and facilitate community decision. Ample information which is a crucial requirement is contributed through various technical researches and analyzes. Here are some of the helpful tools commonly used by planners to aid them:

1. Key Informant Interviews
2. Libraries, Internet, and Survey Research
3. Census and Statistical Analysis
4. Spatial Analysis with Geographical Information System (GIS) and Global Positioning System (GPS) technologies

Key Institutions

Participating structures are primarily led by the government's local authorities and the official tourism board or council, with the involvement of various NGOs, community and indigenous representatives, development organizations, and the academe.

Case Studies

Cultural and Ecotourism in the Mountainous Regions of Central Asia and in the Himalayas

Tourism is coming to the previously isolated but spectacular mountainous regions of Central Asia, the Hindu Kush and the Himalayas. Closed for so many years to visitors from abroad, it now attracts a growing number of foreign tourists by its unique culture and splendid natural beauty. However, while this influx of tourists is bringing economic opportunities and employment to local populations, helping to promote these little-known regions of the world, it has also brought challenges along with it: to ensure that it is well-managed and that its benefits are shared by all.

As a response to this concern, the Norwegian Government, as well as the UNESCO, organized an interdisciplinary project called the Development of Cultural and Eco-tourism in the Mountainous Regions of Central Asia and the Himalayas project. It aims to establish links and promote cooperation between local communities, national and international NGOs, and tour agencies in order to heighten the role of the local community and involve them fully in the employment opportunities and income-generating activities that tourism can bring.

Project activities include training local tour guides, producing high-quality craft items and promoting home-stays and bed-and-breakfast type accommodation.

As of now, the project is drawing on the expertise of international NGOs and tourism professionals in the seven participating countries, making a practical and positive contribution to alleviating poverty by helping local communities to draw the maximum benefit from their region's tourism potential, while protecting the environmental and cultural heritage of the region concerned.

DARK TOURISM

Dark tourism or Grief tourism is tourism involving travel to sites associated with death and suffering. Thanatourism, derived from the Ancient Greek word thanatos for the personification of death, is associated with dark tourism but refers more specifically to violent death; it is used in fewer contexts than the terms dark tourism and grief tourism.

This includes sites of pilgrimage such the site of St Peter's death in Rome; castles and battlefields such as Culloden near Inverness, Scotland; sites of disaster, either natural or man made such as Ground Zero in New York; prisons now open to the public such as Beaumaris Prison in Anglesey, Wales; and purpose built centers such as the London Dungeon.

One of the most notorious destinations for dark tourism is the Nazi extermination camp at Auschwitz in Poland.

DISASTER TOURISM

Disaster tourism is the act of traveling to a disaster area as a matter of curiosity. The behavior can be a nuisance if it hinders rescue, relief, and recovery operations.

Hurricane Katrina

Disaster tourism took hold in the Greater New Orleans Area in the aftermath of Hurricane Katrina. There are now guided bus tours to neighborhoods that were severely damaged by storm-related flooding. Some local residents have criticized these tours as unethical, because the tour companies are profiting from the misery of their communities and families. The Army Corp of Engineers has noted that traffic from tour buses and other tourist vehicles have interfered with the movement of trucks and other cleanup equipment on single-lane residential roads.

Furthermore, during the first six months after the storm, most of these neighborhoods lacked electricity, phone access, street signs, or access to emergency medical or police assistance. Simply traveling to these neighborhoods was hazardous. For these reasons, organized disaster tours are now banned from two of the most severely damaged areas in the city, the Lower 9th and St. Bernard Parish near the Industrial Canal.

On the other hand, such communities as Gentilly and Lakeview, along the 17th Street Canal, have welcomed organized tour groups as a means to publicize the scale of the destruction and attract more aid to the city. Much of the recovery effort in the New Orleans relies on out-of-state volunteers and donations. Numerous non-profit organization, including Habitat for Humanity International and Catholic Charities, have converged on the city to gut and rebuild homes. There is also a movement by local residents to bring congressmen and other national leaders to the city and view the damage in person, since recovery efforts have been hampered by the failure of many homeowners and businesses to receive claims from their insurance providers.

DRUG TOURISM

Drug tourism is travel for the purpose of obtaining or using drugs for personal use that are unavailable or illegal in one's home jurisdiction. This would include crossing a national border to obtain drugs over the counter that are not sold in one's own country, or traveling to another country in order to obtain or use narcotics that are illegal in one's own country, or even traveling from one U.S. state to another in order to buy alcohol or tobacco more easily (although this last situation is often considered too trivial to qualify as drug tourism). Drug tourism has many legal implications, and persons engaging in it sometimes risk prosecution for drug smuggling or other drug-related charges in their home jurisdictions or in the jurisdictions they are visiting, especially if they bring their purchases home rather than using them abroad.

The act of traveling for the purpose of buying or using drugs is itself a criminal offense in some jurisdictions. Amsterdam is a popular destinations for drug tourists, due to the Dutch government's acceptance of marijuana use and possession. Another Dutch city which is visited frequently by drug tourists is Maastricht because of its position close to the borders of Germany and Belgium.

Other popular destinations include Southeast Asia and South America. Drug tourism thrives because legislation controlling the sale, possession, and use of drugs varies dramatically from one jurisdiction to another.

ECOTOURISM

Ecotourism, also known as ecological tourism, is a form of tourism which appeals to the ecologically and socially conscious. Generally speaking, ecotourism focuses on local culture, wilderness adventures, volunteering, personal growth, and learning new ways to live on the planet; typically involving travel to destinations where flora, fauna, and cultural heritage are the primary attractions.

Responsible ecotourism includes programs that minimize the negative aspects of conventional tourism on the environment, and enhance the cultural integrity of local people. Therefore, in addition to evaluating environmental and cultural factors, an integral part of ecotourism is in the promotion of recycling, energy efficiency, water conservation, and creation of economic opportunities for the local communities.

Many global environmental organizations and aid agencies believe that ecotourism has great potential for sustainable development.

Ideally, ecotourism should satisfy several criteria, such as:

- conservation of biological diversity and cultural diversity, through ecosystem protection
- promotion of sustainable use of biodiversity, by providing jobs to local populations
- sharing of socio-economic benefits with local communities and indigenous people by having their informed consent and participation in the management of ecotourism enterprises.
- increase of environmental & cultural knowledge
- minimization of tourism's own environmental impact
- affordability and lack of waste in the form of luxury
- local culture, flora and fauna being the main attractions

For many countries, ecotourism is not simply a marginal activity to finance protection of the environment but as a major industry of the national economy. For example, in places such as Costa Rica, Ecuador, Nepal, Kenya, Madagascar, and Antarctica, ecotourism represents a significant portion of the gross domestic product and economic activity.

The concept of ecotourism is widely misunderstood, and in practice is often used as a marketing tool to promote tourism that is related to nature. Critics claim that ecotourism as practiced and abused often consists of placing a hotel in a splendid landscape, to the detriment of the ecosystem. According to them, ecotourism must above all sensitize people with the beauty and the fragility of nature. They condemn some operators as "greenwashing" their operations; using the label of "ecotourism" and "green-friendly", while behaving in environmentally irresponsible ways. Although academics disagree about who can be classified as an ecotourist and there is precious little statistical data, some estimate that more than five million ecotourists-the majority of the ecotourist population-come from the United States, with others from Western Europe, Canada, and Australia.

Currently there are various moves to create national and international ecotourism accrediation programs, although the process is also controversial. Ecotourism certificates have been put in place at Costa Rica, although some critics have dismissed these programs as greenwashing.

History

Ecotourism, responsible tourism, and sustainable development have become prevalent concepts since the late 1980s, and ecotourism has experienced arguably the fastest growth of all sub-sectors in the tourism industry. The popularity represents a change in tourist perceptions, increased environmental awareness, and a desire to explore natural environments. Such changes have become a statement affirming one's social identity, educational sophistication, and disposable income as it has about preserving the Amazon rainforest or the Caribbean reef for posterity.

With its great potential for environmental protection, the United Nations celebrated the "International Year of Ecotourism" in 2002.

Criticisms

Definitional Problems and Greenwashing

To approach an understanding of the problem, a clear definition must delineate what is, and is not, ecotourism. Ideally, ecotourism satisfies several general criteria, including the conservation of biological diversity and cultural, diversity through ecosystem protection, promotion of sustainable use of biodiversity, share of socio-economic benefits with local communities through informed consent and participation, increase in environmental and cultural knowledge, affordability and reduced waste, and minimization of its own environmental impact. In such ways, it contributes to the long term benefits to both the environment and local communities.

However, in the continuum of tourism activities that stretch from conventional tourism to ecotourism proper, there has been a lot of contention to the limit at which biodiversity preservation, local socio-economic benefits, and environmental impact can be considered "ecotourism". For this reason, environmentalists, special interest groups, and governments define ccotourism differently. Environmental organizations have generally insisted that ecotourism is nature-based, sustainably managed, conservation supporting, and environmentally educated. The tourist industry and governments, however, focus more on the product aspect, treating ecotourism as equivalent to any sort of tourism based in nature. As a further complication, many terms are used under the rubric of ecotourism. Nature tourism, low impact tourism, green tourism, bio-tourism, ecologically responsible tourism, and others have been used in literature and marketing, although they are not necessary synonymous with ecotourism.

The problems associated with defining ecotourism have led to confusion among tourists and academics alike. Definitional problems are also subject of considerable public controversy and concern because of greenwashing, a trend towards the commercialization of tourism schemes disguised as sustainable, nature based, and environmentally friendly ecotourism. According to McLaren, these schemes are environmentally destructive, economically exploitative, and culturally insensitive at its worst. They are also morally disconcerting because they mislead tourists and manipulate their concerns for the environment. Despite objections, greenwashing continues to grow unabated. The Nature's Sacred Paradise, a theme park in Quintana Roo, Mexico, is responsible for displacing local Mayan communities and illegally keeping endangered species in captivity to attract visitors. The development and success of such large scale, energy intensive, and ecologically unsustainable schemes are a testament to the tremendous profits associated with being labeled as ecotourism.

The Negative Psycho-social Impact of Ecotourism

Ecotourism is the trend towards the commercialization of tourism throughout the nation. This trend has become one of the fastest growing sectors of the tourism industry growing annual 10-15% worldwide (Kamuaro, 2007). Ecotourism was first introduced in Africa in the 1950's with the legalization of hunting (Kamuaro, 2007). This need for recreational hunting zones lead to the creation of protected areas, national parks, and game reserves. Today these areas have become important revenue-earning venues with the establishment of lodges and tourist campsites. One definition of ecotourism is "the practice of low-impact, educational, ecologically and culturally sensitive travel that benefits local communities and host countries" (Honey, 1999). Many of the ecotourism projects are not meeting these standards.

Even if some of the guidelines are being executed, the local communities are still facing other negative impacts. South Africa is one of the countries that are reaping significant economic benefits from ecotourism, but negative effects including, physical displacement of persons, gross violation of fundamental rights, and environmental hazards far out weigh the medium-term economic benefits (Kamuaro, 2007). A tremendous amount of money is being spent and human resources continue to be used for ecotourism despite the lack of success stories, and even more money is put into public relation campaigns to dilute the effects of the criticism. Ecotourism channels resources away from other projects that could contribute more sustainable and realistic solutions to pressing social and environmental problems. "The money tourism can generate often ties parks and managements to eco-tourism" (Walpole et al. 2001).

But there is a tension in this relationship because eco-tourism often causes conflict and changes in land-use rights, fails to deliver promises of community-level benefits, damages environments, and has plenty of other social impacts. Indeed many argue repeatedly that eco-tourism is neither ecologically nor socially beneficial, yet it persists as a strategy for conservation and development (West, 2006). While several studies are being done on ways to improve the ecotourism structure, these examples provide reason that it should just stop all together.

The ecotourism system exercises tremendous financial and political influence. The evidence above shows that at the very least a strong case exists for restraining such activities. Funding could be used for field studies aimed at finding alternative solutions to tourism and the diverse problems Africa faces in result of urbanization, industrialization, and over exploitation of agriculture (Kamuaro, 2007). At the local level ecotourism has become a source of conflict over control of land, resources, and tourism profits. There are many problems with the idea of ecotourism. Environmental, the effects on the local people, and conflicts over profit distribution are only a few of the negative effects of ecotourism. In a perfect world more efforts would be made towards educating tourists of the environmental and social effects of their travels. Very few regulations or laws stand in place as boundaries for the investors in ecotourism. These should be implemented to prohibit the promotion of unsustainable ecotourism projects and materials which project false images of destinations, demeaning local and indigenous cultures.

Direct Environmental Impacts

Ecotourism operations typically fail to live up to conservation ideals. It is often overlooked that ecotourism is a highly consumer-centered activity, and that environmental conservation is only a means to further economic growth.

Although ecotourism is intended for small groups, even a modest increase in population, however temporary, puts extra pressure on the local environment and necessitates the development of additional infrastructure and amenities. The construction of water treatment plants, sanitation facilities, and lodges come with the exploitation of non-renewable energy sources and the utilization of already limited local resources. The conversion of natural land to such tourist infrastructure is implicated in deforestation and habitat deterioration of butterflies in Mexico and squirrel monkeys in Costa Rica. In other cases, the environment suffers because local communities are unable to meet the infrastructure demands of ecotourism. The lack of adequate sanitation facilities in many East African parks results in the disposal of campsite sewage in rivers, contaminating the wildlife, livestock, and people who draw drinking water from it.

Aside from environmental degradation with tourist infrastructure, population pressures from ecotourism also leaves behind garbage and pollution associated with the Western lifestyle. Although ecotourists claim to be educationally sophisticated and environmentally concerned, they rarely understand the ecological consequences of their visits and how their day-to-day activities append physical impacts on the environment.

As one scientist observes, they "rarely acknowledge how the meals they eat, the toilets they flush, the water they drink, and so on, are all part of broader regional economic and ecological systems they are helping to reconfigure with their very activities." Nor do ecotourists recognize the great consumption of non-renewable energy required to arrive at their destination, which is typically more remote than conventional tourism destinations. For instance, an exotic journey to a place 10,000 kilometers away consumes about 700 liters of fuel per person.

Ecotourism activities are, in of itself, issues in environmental impact because they disturb fauna and flora. Ecotourists believe that because they are only taking pictures and leaving footprints, they keep ecotourism sites pristine, but even harmless sounding activities such as a nature hike can be ecologically destructive.

In the Annapurna Circuit in Nepal, ecotourists have worn down the marked trails and created alternate routes, contributing to soil impaction, erosion, and plant damage. Where the ecotourism activity involves wildlife viewing, it can scare away animals, disrupt their feeding and nesting sites, or acclimate them to the presence of people. In Kenya, disruption of wildlife observers drive cheetahs off their reserves, increasing the risk of inbreeding and further endangering the species.

Environmental Hazards

We already understand that biodiversity and environmentally intact lands form the basis of ecological stability. Unfortunately, industrialization, urbanization, and unsustainable agriculture practices have all had serious effects on the environment. Ecotourism is now also playing a role in this depletion. While the term ecotourism may sound relatively benign, one of its most serious impacts is its consumption of virgin territories (Kamuaro, 2007). These invasions often include deforestation, disruption of ecological life systems and various forms of pollution, all of which contribute to environmental degradation. The number of motor vehicles crossing the park increases as tour drivers search for rare species.

The number of roads has disrupted the grass cover which has serious effects on plant and animal species. These areas also have a higher rate of disturbances and invasive species because of all the traffic moving off the beaten path into new undiscovered areas (Kamuaro, 2007). Ecotourism also has an affect on species through the value placed on them. "Certain species have gone from being little known or valued by local people to being highly valued commodities.

The commodification of plants may erase their social value and lead to overproduction within protected areas. Local people and their images can also be turned into commodities" (West, 2006). Kamuaro brings up a relatively obvious contradiction, any commercial venture into unspoiled, pristine land with or without the "eco" prefix as a contradiction in terms. To generate revenue you have to have a high number of traffic, tourists, which inevitably means a higher pressure on the environment.

Local Peoples

Most forms of ecotourism are owned by foreign investors and corporations that provide few benefits to local communities. An overwhelming majority of profits are put into the pockets of investors instead of reinvestment into the local economy or environmental protection. The limited numbers of local people who are employed in the economy enter at its lowest level, and are unable to live in tourist areas because of meager wages and a two market system. In some cases, the resentment by local people results in environmental degradation. As a highly publicized case, the Maasai nomads in Kenya killed wildlife in national parks to show aversion to unfair compensation terms and displacement from traditional lands. The lack of economic opportunities for local people also constrains them to degrade the environment as a means of sustenance. The presence of affluent ecotourists encourage the development of destructive markets in wildlife souvenirs, such as the sale of coral trinkets on tropical islands and animal products in Asia, contributing to illegal harvesting and poaching from the environment. In Surinam, sea turtle reserves use a large portion of their budget to guard against these activities.

Displacement of People

One of the most powerful examples of communities being moved in order to create a park is the story of the Masai. About 70% of national parks and game reserves in East Africa are on Masai land (Kamuaro, 2007). The first undesirable impact of tourism was that of the extent of land lost from the Masai culture. Local and national governments took advantage of the Masai's ignorance on the situation and robbed them of huge chunks of grazing land, putting to risk their only socioeconomic livelihood. In Kenya the Masai also have not gained any economic benefits. Despite lose of their land, employment favors better educated workers. Further more the investors in this area are not local and have not put profits back into local economy. In some cases game reserves can be created without informing or consulting local people, who come to find out about the situation when an eviction notice is delivered (Kamuaro, 2007).

Another source of resentment is the manipulation of the local people by their government. "Eco-tourism works to create simplistic images of local people and their uses and understandings of their surroundings. Through the lens of these simplified images, officials direct policies and projects towards the local people and the local people are blamed if the projects fail" (West, 2006). Clearly tourism as a trade is not empowering the local people who make it rich and satisfying. Instead ecotourism exploits and depletes, particularly in African Masai tribes. It has to be reoriented to serve useful to local communities and to become sustainable.

Threats to Indigenous Cultures

Ecotourism often claims that it preserves and "enhances" local cultures. However, evidence shows that with the establishment of protected areas local people have illegally lost their homes, and most often with no compensation (Kamuaro, 2007). What about pushing people onto marginal lands with harsh climates, poor soils, lack of water, and infested with livestock and disease is "enhancing"? The establishment of parks does nothing but create harsh survival realities and deprives the people of their traditional use of land and natural resources. Ethnic groups are increasingly being seen as a "backdrop" to the scenery and wildlife. The local people struggle for cultural survival and freedom of cultural expression while being "observed" by tourists. Local indigenous people also have strong resentment towards the change, "Tourism has been allowed to develop with virtually no controls. Too many lodges have been built, too much firewood is being used and no limits are being placed on tourism vehicles. They regularly drive off-track and harass the wildlife. Their vehicle tracks crisscross the entire Masai Mara. Inevitably the bush is becoming eroded and degraded" (Kamuaro, 2007).

Mismanagement of Ecotourism Sites

While governments are typically entrusted with the administration and enforcement of environmental protection, they often lack the commitment or capability to manage ecotourism sites effectively. The regulations for environmental protection may be vaguely defined, costly to implement, hard to enforce, and uncertain in effectiveness. Government regulatory agencies, as political bodies, are susceptible to making decisions that spend budget on politically beneficial but environmentally unproductive projects. Because of prestige and conspicuousness, the construction of an attractive visitor's center at an ecotourism site may take precedence over more pressing environmental concerns like acquiring habitat, protecting endemic species, and removing invasive ones. Finally, influential groups can pressure and sway the interests of the government to their favor. The government and its regulators can become vested in the benefits of the ecotourism industry which they are supposed to regulate, causing restrictive environmental regulations and enforcement to become more lenient.

Management of ecotourism sites by private ecotourism companies offers an alternative to the cost of regulation and deficiency of government agencies. It is believed that these companies have a self interest in limited environmental degradation, because tourists will pay more for pristine environments, which translates to higher profit. However, theory indicates that this practice is not economically feasible and will fail to manage the environment.

The model of monopolistic competition states that distinctiveness will entail profits, but profits will promote imitation. A company that protects its ecotourism sites is able to charge a premium for the novel experience and pristine environment. But when other companies view the success of this approach, they also enter the market with similar practices, increasing competition and reducing demand. Eventually, the demand will be reduced until the economic profit is zero. A cost-benefit analysis shows that the company bears the cost of environmental protection without receiving the gains. Without economic incentive, the whole premise of self interest through environmental protection is quashed; instead, ecotourism companies will minimize environment related expenses and maximize tourism demand.

The tragedy of the commons offers another model for economic unsustainability from environmental protection, in ecotourism sites utilized by many companies. Although there is a communal incentive to protect the environment, maximizing the benefits in the long run, a company will conclude that it is in their best interest to utilize the ecotourism site beyond its sustainable level. By increasing the number of ecotourists, for instance, a company gains all the economic benefit while paying only a part of the environmental cost. In the same way, a company recognizes that there is no incentive to actively protect the environment; they bear all the costs, while the benefits are shared by all other companies. The result, again, is mismanagement.

Taken together, the mobility of foreign investment and lack of economic incentive for environmental protection means that ecotourism companies are disposed to establishing themselves in new sites once their existing one is sufficiently degraded.

IMPROVING SUSTAINABILITY

Regulation and Accreditation

Because the regulation of ecotourism is poorly implemented or nonexistent, ecologically destructive greenwashed operations like underwater hotels, helicopter tours, and wildlife theme parks are categorized as ecotourism along with canoeing, camping, photography, and wildlife observation. The failure to acknowledge responsible, low impact ecotourism puts these companies at a competitive disadvantage.

Many environmentalists have argued for a global standard of accreditation, differentiating ecotourism companies based on their level of environmental commitment. A national or international regulatory board would enforce accreditation procedures, with representation from various groups including governments, hotels, tour operators, travel agents, guides, airlines, local authorities, conservation organizations, and non-governmental organizations. The decisions of the board would be sanctioned by governments, so that non-compliant companies would be legally required to disassociate themselves from the use of the ecotourism brand.

Crinion suggests a Green Stars System based on criteria including a management plan, benefit for the local community, small group interaction, education value, and staff training. Ecotourists who consider their choices would be confident of a genuine ecotourism experience when they see the higher star rating. In addition, environmental impact assessments could be used as a form of accreditation. Feasibility is evaluated from a scientific basis, and recommendations could be made to optimally plan infrastructure, set tourist capacity, and manage the ecology. This form of accreditation is more sensitive to site specific conditions.

Guidelines and Education for Ecotourists

An environmental protection strategy must address the issue of ecotourists removed from the cause-and-effect of their actions on the environment. More initiatives should be carried out to improve their awareness, sensitize them to environmental issues, and care about the places they visit.

Tour guides are an obvious and direct medium to communicate awareness. With the confidence of ecotourists and intimate knowledge of the environment, they can actively discuss conservation issues. A tour guide training program in Costa Rica's Tortuguero National Park has helped mitigate negative environmental impacts by providing information and regulating tourists on the parks' beaches used by nesting endangered sea turtles.

Small Scale, Slow Growth, Locally based Ecotourism

The underdevelopment theory of tourism describes a new form of imperialism by multinational corporations that control ecotourism resources. These corporations finance and profit from the development of large scale ecotourism that causes excessive environmental degradation, loss of traditional culture and way of life, and exploitation of local labor. In Zimbabwe and Nepal's Annapurna region, where underdevelopment is taking place, more than 90 percent of ecotourism revenues are expatriated to the parent countries, and less than 5 percent go into local communities.

The lack of sustainability highlights the need for small scale, slow growth, and locally based ecotourism. Local peoples have a vested interest in the well being of their community, and are therefore more accountable to environmental protection than multinational corporations. The lack of control, westernization, adverse impacts to the environment, loss of culture and traditions outweigh the benefits of establishing large scale ecotourism.

The increased contributions of communities to locally managed ecotourism create viable economic opportunities, including high level management positions, and reduce environmental issues associated with poverty and unemployment. Because the ecotourism experience is marketed to a different lifestyle from large scale ecotourism, the development of facilities and infrastructure does not need to conform to corporate Western tourism standards, and can be much simpler and less expensive. There is a greater multiplier effect on the economy, because local products, materials, and labor are used. Profits accrue locally, and import leakages are reduced. However, even this form of tourism may require foreign investment for promotion or start up. When such investments are required, it is cruical for communities for find a company or non-governmental organization that reflects the philosophy of ecotourism; sensitive to their concerns and willing to cooperate at the expense of profit.

The basic assumption of the multiplier effect is that the economy starts off with unused resources, for example, that many workers are cyclically unemployed and much of industrial capacity is sitting idle or incompletely utilized. By increasing demand in the economy it is then possible to boost production. If the economy was already at full employment, with only structural, frictional, or other supply-side types of unemployment, any attempt to boost demand would only lead to inflation. For various laissez-faire schools of economics which embrace Say's Law and deny the possibility of Keynesian inefficiency and under-employment of resources, therefore, the multiplier concept is irrelevant or wrong-headed.

As an example, consider the government increasing its expenditure on roads by $1 million, without a corresponding increase in taxation. This sum would go to the road builders, who would hire more workers and distribute the money as wages and profits. The households receiving these incomes will save part of the money and spend the rest on consumer goods. These expenditures in turn will generate more jobs, wages, and profits, and so on with the income and spending circulating around the economy.

The multiplier effect arises because of the induced increases in consumer spending which occur due to the increased incomes—and because of the feedback into increasing business revenues, jobs, and income again. This process does not lead to an economic explosion not only because of the supply-side barriers at potential output (full employment) but because at each "round", the increase in consumer spending is less than the increase in consumer incomes. That is, the marginal propensity to consume (mpc) is less than one, so that each round some extra income goes into saving, leaking out of the cumulative process. Each increase in spending is thus smaller than that of the previous round, preventing an explosion.

EXTREME TOURISM

Extreme tourism or shock tourism is a type of niche tourism involving travel to dangerous places (mountains, jungles, deserts, caves, etc.) or participation in dangerous events. Extreme tourism overlaps with extreme sport. The two share the main attraction, "adrenaline rush" caused by an element of risk, and differing mostly in the degree of engagement and professionalism.

Extreme tourism is a growing business in the countries of the former Soviet Union (Russia, Ukraine, Armenia, etc.) and in South American countries like Peru, Chile and Argentina. The mountainous and rugged terrain of Northern Pakistan has also developed into a popular extreme tourism location.

While traditional tourism requires significant investments in hotels, roads, etc., extreme tourism requires much less to jump-start a business. In addition to traditional travel-based tourism destinations, various exotic attractions are suggested, such as flyovers in MiGs at 2.5 Mach, ice diving in the White Sea, or travelling across the Chernobyl zone.

FEMALE SEX TOURISM

Female sex tourism is travel by women, partially or fully for the purpose of having sex.

Overview

Female sex tourism differs from male sex tourism in that women do not use bars, sex shows and formal tours to meet foreign men. There are "de facto" tours, however, such as airplanes bound to the Gambia in West Africa full of British and Scandinavian women seeking affairs with beach boys.

Often such trips are referred to by women as "romance tourism."

Women usually give clothes, meals, cash and gifts to their male prostitutes. In some destinations, there are "going rates" for male companionship, ranging from $50 to $200. In few destinations, especially in Southern Europe, Turkey, Bali and the French Caribbean, men do not expect to be compensated.

Destinations

While men tend to go to Asia for sex tourism, women tend to head to the Caribbean, Southern Europe, and Africa. The patterns have been explored by Michel Houellebecq in Platform and in the non-fiction work Romance on the Road, and are important in that they support the idea that sex tourism by both men and women reflects serious problems in the tourists' home countries, including a dating war, or profound conflict between the sexes.

Thailand, the Dominican Republic and Cuba are exceptional in that both male and female sex tourists find these places all-purpose sexual emporia.

The primary destinations for female sex tourism are Southern Europe (mainly Italy, Greece, Turkey, Croatia and Spain), the Caribbean (led by Jamaica, Barbados and the Dominican Republic), Ghana and Kenya in Africa, Bali in Indonesia and Phuketin Thailand. Lesser destinations include Nepal, Morocco, Fiji, Ecuador and Costa Rica.

Lesbian sex tourism is nascent but evident in Lesbos (Mytilini) in Greece; Bangkok and Pattaya in Thailand, and on Bali in Indonesia.

Terms used for Female Sex Tourists

Tourist women are called Shirley Valentines (if British), longtails (in Bermuda), yellow cabs (Japan) and, in Jamaica, milk bottles if newly arrived or Stellas if black. Female sex tourism in Barbados has been dubbed "Canadian secretary syndrome."

The men who chase tourist women are kamakia ("fishing harpoons," Greece),galebovi ("seagulls,"Croatia), sharks (Costa Rica), rent-a-dreads, rent-a-rastas, rent-a-gents and the Foreign Service (Caribbean), Kuta Cowboys or pemburu-bule ("whitey hunters," Bali), Marlboro men (Jordan), bomsas or bumsters (the Gambia), sanky pankies (Dominican Republic), "gringa hunter" in Ecuador and "brichero" in Peru.

History

Barring some isolated cases of women traveling for sex among North American Indian tribes and within Turkey, female travel sex (involving American and English women) began in Rome in the late 1840s, at the same time as feminism's first wave, which encouraged independence and travel. Affairs and intrigues, particularly between American heiresses and down-on their luck European aristocrats, continued steadily until World War I and inspired Henry James's Daisy Miller, Joaquin Miller's The One Fair Woman, and much of the early output of E.M. Forster. Female sex travel declined from the time of the Depression until the 1960s, with the exception of India, Nepal and Thailand, where intrepid women from England, France, Czechoslovakia, the United States and elsewhere continued to attract the attention of maharajas and other Asian royals, despite the uproar of World War II.

Coincident with the explosion of leisure travel in the 1960s and feminism's second wave, sex tourism by women re-ignited, first via French Canadian women traveling to Barbados and Swedish and Northern European women to Spain, Greece, Yugoslavia and the Gambia. Female sex travel became ubiquitous throughout the Caribbean, from the tiniest islands through the big destinations of Jamaica, the Dominican Republic and Barbados. In the 1990s, women from Japan and Taiwan began to appear on the beaches of Bali and Phuket in Thailand.

Today, many other destinations are popular, including Morocco, Nepal, Thailand, Ecuador, Costa Rica, Mexico—everywhere with beaches (or in Nepal's case, mountains) and a surplus of underemployed men.

Reasons

Female sex tourism's first and second waves coincided not only with feminism but with Victorian-era man shortages that began in England and later cropped in continental Europe and the United States. Other societal reasons for women seeking intimate companionship abroad include the dating war, as typified by extreme competition between the sexes in schools, the workplace, while dating, in marriages, and even in contentious divorces. The dating war appears to especially drive sex tourism by Australian and Japanese women, and to a lesser extent, German and Scandinavian female tourists.

Another factor in women engaging in holiday romance is identity loss. Many women behave while traveling in a way at odds to how they behave at home, where fear of the "slut" label curbs the kind of hedonistic behavior seen on holiday. Traveling and expatriate women often try on a new, more experimental identity when away from family and friends.

Additional reasons include:

- sexual connoisseurship—an interest in experiencing a variety of men
- a search for healing after a divorce or breakup (see Michelle Thomas, in Major academic publications, below)
- prolonged involuntary celibacy
- the commodification of sex, whereby affection is now something that can be purchased by women, as well as men, as well as the globalization of sex and affection markets
- interest in fulfilling sexual fantasies

Depictions

Non-fiction books include Anne Cumming's The Love Habit and The Love Quest, Fiona Pitt-Kethley's The Pan Principle and Journeys to the Underworld, Cleo Odzer's Patpong Sisters and Lucretia Stewart's The Weather Prophet.

Female sex tourists have been notoriously difficult to find and interview on the record (see de Albuquerque, 1998, in "Major academic publications" subheading, below). Thus some observers have turned to film and fiction to examine the motivations of women who travel for sex, love and affection. Movies include Heading South (Vers le Sud), with Charlotte Rampling which depicts three Western tourists in Haiti in the 1970s, taking their pleasure with local men. Earlier film depictions include How Stella Got Her Groove Back and Shirley Valentine. Stella led to a quantifiable increase in trips by women to Jamaica, according to Michele Faul's Associated Press article, 12/6/1998, " 'Stella' the Movie Attracting Single Women to Jamaica."

SEX TOURISM

Sex tourism is travel to engage in sexual intercourse or sexual activity with prostitutes, and is typically undertaken internationally by tourists from wealthier countries whose payment for services may then be rendered either in cash or in kind.

The World Tourism Organization, a specialized agency of the United Nations, defines sex tourism as "trips organized from within the tourism sector, or from outside this sector but using its structures and networks, with the primary purpose of effecting a commercial sexual relationship by the tourist with residents at the destination". The U.N. opposes sex tourism citing health, social and cultural consequences for both tourist home countries and destination countries, especially in situations exploiting gender, age, social and economic inequalities in sex tourism destinations.

Attractions for sex tourists can include reduced costs for services in the destination country, along with either legal prostitution or indifferent law enforcement and access to child prostitution.

Destinations

National destinations for sex tourists include Thailand, Brazil, Dominican Republic, Costa Rica, and Cuba. An individual city or region can have a particular reputation as a sex tourist destination. Many of these coincide with major red-light districts, and include Amsterdam in the Netherlands; Zona Norte in Tijuana, Mexico; Bangkok, Pattaya and Phuket in Thailand; Vladivostok in Russian Far East, destination for Japanese sex tourists, and Angeles City, the site of a former United States military base in the province of Pampanga, Philippines. In the United States, prostitution is largely illegal, with the exception of rural areas of the state of Nevada; these have become a sex tourist destination for some Americans. To a lesser extent, several other large cities in the U.S. are also domestic sex tourist destinations despite legal sanctions on prostitution.

Conversely, prostitution is a legal activity in a growing list of other nations worldwide including in many of these destinations.

Female Sex Tourism Destinations

The primary destinations for female sex tourism are Southern Europe (mainly Italy, former Yugoslavia, Turkey, Greece and Spain), the Caribbean (led by Jamaica, Barbados and the Dominican Republic), parts of Africa, Pattaya or Phuket in Thailand. Lesser destinations include Nepal, Morocco, Fiji, Ecuador and Costa Rica. Female sex tourism differs from male sex tourism, in that women do not usually go to specific bars. Women usually give clothes, meals, cash and gifts to their prostitutes, but not all (especially in Southern Europe) expect compensation.

Criminality and Controversy

Tourism Involving Sex with Minors

Child Wise defines child sex tourism as "the commercial sexual exploitation of children by foreigners", usually referring to:

- travel to other countries to engage in sexual acts with children, or
- foreigners engaging in sexual activity with children while overseas

While most sex tourists only engage in this activity with other adults, some actively look for child prostitutes, while others are not very selective either way regarding age. The

WTO makes a distinction between "sex tourism" and "child sex tourism." A tourist who has sex with a child prostitute offends the spirit of the international Convention on the Rights of the Child and the Optional protocol on the sale of children, child prostitution and child pornography, and, in addition to breaking the law in the host country, might well also be doing so in the country the tourist is a national of. A growing number of countries are enacting laws with extra-territorial reach in order to meet their obligations under the covenants above, and consequently punishing citizens who engage in sex with minors whilst overseas. But being difficult to police and enforce these crimes continue nonetheless.

The term "child" is often used as defined by the international conventions above and refers to any person below the age of consent. Many countries have signed the Worst Forms of Child Labour Convention, 1999 and implemented domestic law making having sex with child prostitutes a criminal offence for their nationals or inhabitants including when practised abroad regardless of whether it is forbidden by the laws of the destination country. Singapore has been criticized for having no such law, in spite of being adjacent to the sex tourism destination of Batam in Indonesia, which has many underage sex workers, many of whom have been forced into prostitution.

In 2004 Canada started to prosecute individuals under the sex tourism law. The first individual charged in Canada under this law was Donald Bakker. Australia has long done so: with a conviction in 1996 after enactment of legislation in 1994. Its Government has, for example, caused an international political incident in pressing for the extradition of suspended Solomon Islands Attorney-General Julian Moti, an Australian citizen, to face possible charges over alleged offences dating back to 1997. According to the Cambodia minister for Woman's Affairs, it is not tourists who are the prime culprits of pedophilia in her country, but the locals.

Legal Issues in the United States

Federal law (see PROTECT Act of 2003) prohibits United States citizens or permanent residents to engage in international travel with the purpose or effect of having commercial sex with a person under the age of 18, or any sex with a person under the age of 16; facilitating such travel is also illegal. Arrests by Immigration and Customs Enforcement are becoming common, however prosecutions under this law are still very rare.

As of 2005, there has been one effort to prosecute a sex tour operator: Big Apple Oriental Tours of New York was prosecuted for "promotion of prostitution" by the New York State Attorney General after lobbying by feminist human rights groups, however the case has been thrown out twice.

HR 972, the Trafficking Victims Protection Reauthorization Act of 2005 reauthorizes the 2000 law, but it also gives U.S. law enforcement better tools to study human trafficking within the United States and to prosecute those who purchase sex acts. The measure authorizes $50 million for grants to state and local law enforcement to investigate and prosecute persons who engage in the purchase of commercial sex acts.

Scandals

In 2005 it was reported that Philippe Servaty, a newspaper columnist for Le Soir, traveled to Morocco where he persuaded women to engage in sexual activity by promising to marry and bring them to Belgium. He then posted photos online to boast of his conquests, but when his explicit materials were circulated back to Morocco many of the women were arrested, had their lives ruined, committed suicide or disappeared.

Academic Study

University of Leicester sociologists studied this subject as part of a research project for the Economic and Social Research Council and End Child Prostitution and Trafficking campaign. The study included interviews with over 250 Caribbean sex tourists. Among their findings:

- Preconceptions about race and gender influenced their opinions.
- Economically underdeveloped tourist-receiving countries are promoted as being culturally different so

that (in the Western tourist's understanding) prostitution and traditional male domination of women have less stigma than similar practices might have in their home countries.

Documentaries

Canadian film makers have been active at reporting on sex tourism. Documentary titles include:

- Falang: Behind Bangkok's Smile by Jordon Clark (2005) (this title at the Internet Movie Database), set in Thailand
- the CBC series, the Lens episode "Selling Sex in Heaven" (2005) (this title at the Internet Movie Database), set in the Philippines.
- Channel 4 Cutting Edge episode "The Child Sex Trade" (2003), set in Romania, Italy

Depictions in Fiction and Popular Culture

- The 2005 film Heading South describes the experiences of a group of middle-aged women in the late 1970s, who travel to Haiti for the purposes of sexual tourism.
- In the animated TV series South Park the character Chef joins the Super Adventure Club which travels the world having sex with children.
- Sex tourism is a major theme of Platform, a novel by Michel Houellebecq.
- In the 2005 film Hostel, directed by Eli Roth, depicts sex tourism in Slovakia
- The film Macho Dancer deals with male sex workers in Manila. It includes characters who are female prostitutes.

TRAFFICKING IN HUMAN BEINGS

Trafficking of human beings is the recruitment, transportation, transfer, harbouring or receipt of people for the purpose of exploitation. Trafficking involves a process of using illicit means such as threat, use of force, or other forms of coercion, of abduction, of fraud, of deception, of the abuse of power or of a position of vulnerability.

Exploitation includes forcing people into prostitution or other forms of sexual exploitation, forced labour or services, slavery or practices similar to slavery, servitude or the removal of organs. For children exploitation may include also, illicit international adoption, trafficking for early marriage, recruitment as child soldiers, for begging or for sports (such as child camel jockeys or football players), or for recruitment for religious cults.

Overview

Human trafficking differs from people smuggling. In the latter, people voluntarily request smuggler's service for fees and there may be no deception involved in the (illegal) agreement. On arrival at their destination, the smuggled person is usually free. On the other hand, the trafficking victim is enslaved, or the terms of their debt bondage are fraudulent or highly exploitative. The trafficker takes away the basic human rights of the victim. Victims are sometimes tricked and lured by false promises or physically forced. Some traffickers use coercive and manipulative tactics including deception, intimidation, feigned love, isolation, threat and use of physical force, debt bondage, other abuse, or even force-feeding with drugs to control their victims.

In the case of children, such practices are considered child trafficking even if none of the illicit means previously described are used.

Trafficked people usually come from the poorer regions of the world, where opportunities are limited, and are often from the most vulnerable in society, such as runaways, refugees, or other displaced persons, (though they may come from any social background, class or race. People who are seeking entry to other countries may be picked up by traffickers, and-typically-misled into thinking that they will be free after being smuggled across the border. In some cases, they are captured through slave raiding, although this is increasingly rare.

Trafficking of children often involves exploitation of the parents' extreme poverty. The latter may sell children to traffickers in order to pay off debts or gain income or they may be deceived concerning the prospects of training and a better life for their children. In West Africa, trafficked children have often lost one or both parents to the African AIDS crisis.

Women, who form over 80% of trafficking victims, are particularly at risk to become involved in sex trafficking. Potential kidnappers exploit lack of opportunities, promise good jobs or opportunities for study, and then force the victims to become prostitutes, participate in pornography or escort services. Through agents and brokers who arrange the travel and job placements, women are escorted to their destinations and delivered to the employers. Upon reaching their destinations, some women learn that they have been deceived about the nature of the work they will do; most have been lied to about the financial arrangements and conditions of their employment; and all find themselves in coercive and abusive situations from which escape is both difficult and dangerous.

The main motive of a woman (in some cases an underage girl) to accept an offer from a trafficker is better financial opportunities for herself or her family. In many cases traffickers initially offer 'legitimate' work or the promise of an opportunity to study. The main types of work offered are in the catering and hotel industry, in bars and clubs, modeling contracts, or au pair work. Offers of marriage are sometimes used by traffickers as well as threats, intimidation and kidnapping. In the majority of cases, the women end up in prostitution. Also some (migrating) prostitutes become victims of human trafficking. Some women know they will be working as prostitutes, but they have a too-rosy picture of the circumstances and the conditions of the work in the country of destination.

Men are also at risk of being trafficked for unskilled work predominantly involving hard labor. Other forms of trafficking include bonded and sweatshop labor, forced marriage, and domestic servitude. Children are also trafficked for both labor exploitation and sexual exploitation. On a related issue, children are forced to be child soldiers.

Many women are forced into the sex trade after answering false advertisements, and others are simply kidnapped. Thousands of children from Asia, Africa, and South America are sold into the global sex trade every year. Often they are kidnapped or orphaned, and sometimes they are actually sold by their own families.

Extent

United States State Department data "estimated 600,000 to 820,000 men, women, and children [are] trafficked across international borders each year, approximately 80 percent are women and girls and up to 50 percent are minors. The data also illustrate that the majority of transnational victims are trafficked into commercial sexual exploitation." Due to the illegal nature of trafficking and differences in methodology, the exact extent is unknown.

An estimated 14,000 people are trafficked into the United States each year, although again because trafficking is illegal, accurate statistics are difficult. According to the Massachusetts based Trafficking Victims Outreach and Services Networkin Massachusetts alone, there were 55 documented cases of human trafficking in 2005 and the first half of 2006 in Massachusetts. In 2004, the Royal Canadian Mounted Police (RCMP) estimated that 600-800 persons are trafficked into Canada annually and that additional 1,500-2,200 persons are trafficked through Canada into the United States.

In the United Kingdom, 71 women were known to have been trafficked into prostitution in 1998 and the Home Office recognized that the scale is likely greater as the problem is hidden and research estimates that the actual figure could be up to 1,420 women trafficked into the UK during the same period. Trafficking in people is increasing in Africa, South Asia and into North America.

Russia is a major source of women trafficked globally for the purpose of sexual exploitation. Annually, thousands of Russian women end up as prostitutes in China, Japan or South Korea. Russia is also a significant destination and transit country for persons trafficked for sexual and labor exploitation from regional and neighboring countries into Russia, and on to the Gulf states, Europe, Asia, and North America. The ILO estimates that 20 percent of the five million illegal immigrants in Russia are victims of forced labor, which is a form of trafficking. There were reports of trafficking of children and of child sex tourism in Russia. The Government of Russia has made some effort to combat trafficking but has also been criticized for not complying with the minimum standards for the elimination of trafficking.

The majority of child trafficking cases are in Asia, although it is a global problem. In Thailand, non-governmental organisations (NGO) have estimated that up to a third of prostitutes are children under 18, many trafficked from outside Thailand. In Ukraine, a survey conducted by the NGO "La Strada-Ukraine" in 2001-2003, based on a sample of 106 women being trafficked out of Ukraine found that 3% were under 18, and the US State Department reported in 2004 that incidents of minors being trafficked was increasing.

In Asia, Japan is the major destination country for trafficked women, especially from the Philippines and Thailand. The US State Department has rated Japan as either a 'Tier 2' or a 'Tier 2 Watchlist' country every year since 2001 in its annual Trafficking in Persons reports. Both these ratings implied that Japan was (to a greater or lesser extent) not fully compliant with minimum standards for the elimination of human trafficking trade.

In Ukraine, a survey conducted by the NGO "La Strada-Ukraine" in 2001-2003, based on a sample of 106 women being trafficked out of Ukraine found that 3% were under 18, and the US State Department reported in 2004 that incidents of minors being trafficked was increasing.

In the United Kingdom, Vietnamese human trafficking have been discovered in the past few years. Many Vietnamese people are trafficked to work in illegal Vietnamese cannabis factories throughout the country, as the recent police Operation Keymer showed. Another recent police Operation Pentameter discovered illegal Vietnamese are also smuggled in to work in Vietnamese nail salons. Recently the UK authority planned to deport over 500 children back to Vietnam who had been smuggled into the country.

Reporters have witnessed a rapid increase in prostitution in Cambodia, Bosnia, and Kosovo after UN and, in the case of the latter two, NATO peacekeeping forces moved in. Peacekeeping forces have been linked to trafficking and forced prostitution. Proponents of peacekeeping argue that the actions of a few should not incriminate the many participants in the mission, yet NATO and the UN have come under criticism for not taking the issue of forced prostitution linked to peacekeeping missions seriously enough.

In the western world, Canada in particular has a major problem with modern-day sexual slavery. In a 2006 report the Future Group, a Canadian humanitarian organization dedicated to ending human trafficking, ranked eight industrialized nations and gave Canada an F for its "abysmal" record treating victims. The report, titled "Falling Short of the Mark: An International Study on the Treatment of Human Trafficking Victims", concluded that Canada "is an international embarrassment" when it comes to combatting this form of slavery.

The report's principal author Benjamin Perrin wrote, "Canada has ignored calls for reform and continues to re-traumatize trafficking victims, with few exceptions, by subjecting them to routine deportation and fails to provide even basic support services."

In the report, the only other country to flunk was the United Kingdom, which received a D, while the United States received a B+ and Australia, Norway, Sweden, Germany and Italy all received grades of B or B-. The report criticizes former Liberal Party of Canada cabinet ministers Irwin Cotler, Joe Volpe and Pierre Pettigrew for "passing the buck" on the issue. Commenting on the report, the then Minister of Citizenship and Immigration, Monte Solberg told Sun Media Corporation, "It's very damning, and if there are obvious legislative or regulatory fixes that need to be done, those have to become priorities, given especially that we're talking about very vulnerable people."

Cause of Trafficking

Some causes of trafficking include:

- poverty
- perceived higher standards of life elsewhere
- lack of employement opportunities
- organised crime and presence of organised criminal gangs
- regional imbalances
- economic disparities
- social discrimination
- corruption in governement
- political instability
- armed conflict
- uprooting of communities because of mega projects without proper Resttlement and Rehabilitation packages.
- Profitability
- Growing deprivation and marginalization of the poor
- Insufficient penalties against traffickers
- According to the UN a major factor that has allowed the growth of sexual trafficking is "Governments and human rights organizations alike have simply judged the woman guilty of prostitution and minimized the trafficker's role."
- Driven by demand; demand is high for prostitutes and other forms of labor in host countries; therefore there is a very profitable market available to those who wish to become handlers.

Trafficking in people has been facilitated by porous borders and advanced communication technologies, it has become increasingly transnational in scope and highly lucrative. Unlike drugs or arms, people can be "sold" many times. The opening up of Asian markets, porous borders, the end of the Soviet

Union and the collapse of the former Yugoslavia have contributed to this globalization.

Government Action against Human Trafficking

A human trafficking awareness poster from the Canadian Department of Justice Actions taken to combat human trafficking vary from government to government. Some have introduced legislation specifically aimed at making human trafficking illegal. Governments can also develop systems of co-operation between different nation's law enforcement agencies and with non-government organisations (NGOs). Other actions governments could take is raise awareness. This can take on three forms. Firstly in raising awareness amongst potential victims, in particular in countries where human traffickers are active. Secondly, raising awareness amongst police, social welfare workers and immigration officers. And in countries where prostitution is legal or semi-legal, raising awareness amongst the clients of prostitution, to look out for signs of a human trafficking victim. Laws against trafficking in the United States are prosecuted at the federal level. The overwhelming majority of states do not have laws against human trafficking. For example, in Maryland it is a felony to have sex with a minor, but only a misdemeanor for making it available to those who wish to have sex with a minor. Raising awareness can take on different forms. One method is through the use of awareness films or through posters.

Criticism of Bangladesh on Human Trafficking

In June 2006, the government of Bangladesh issued a restraining order preventing Sigma Huda, U.N. special reporter on trafficking in persons, from leaving the country to deliver a key report on trafficking before the Human Rights Council in Geneva on June 11, 2007. U.N. High Commissioner for Human Rights Louise Arbour has asked Bangladesh to clarify corruption charges against a U.N. human rights investigator, which will prevent her from addressing the main U.N. rights body. The Coalition Against Trafficking in Women issued a statement calling this "an outrage and a violation of her right to freedom of movement and freedom of speech."

International Law

In 2000 the United Nations adopted the Convention against Transnational Organized Crime, also called the Palermo Convention and two Palermo protocols thereto:

- Protocol to Prevent, Suppress and Punish Trafficking in Persons, especially Women and Children; and
- Protocol against the Smuggling of Migrants by Land, Sea and Air.

All of these instruments contain elements of the current international law on trafficking in human beings.

Council of Europe

The Council of Europe Convention on Action against Trafficking in Human Beings was adopted by the Council of Europe on 16 May 2005. The aim of the convention is to prevent and combat the trafficking in human beings. Of the 46 members of the Council of Europe, so far 31 have signed the convention and 1 has ratified it.(29 June 2006).

United States Federal Law

The United States federal government has taken a firm stance against human trafficking both within its borders and beyond. Domestically, human trafficking is prosecuted through the Civil Rights Division, Criminal Section of the United States Department of Justice. Older statutes used to protect 13th Amendment rights within United States borders are Title 18 U.S.C., Sections 1581 and 1584. Section 1584 makes it a crime to force a person to work against his will. This compulsion can be effected by use of force, threat of force, threat of legal coercion or by "a climate of fear", that is, an environment wherein individuals believe they may be harmed by leaving or refusing to work. Section 1581 similarly makes it illegal to force a person to work through "debt servitude".

New laws were passed under the Victims of Trafficking and Violence Protection Act of 2000. The new laws responded to a changing face of trafficking in the United States. It allowed for greater statutory maximum sentences for traffickers, provided resources for protection of and assistance for victims of trafficking and created avenues for inter-agency cooperation in the field of human trafficking. It also allows many trafficking victims to remain in the United States and apply for permanent residency. This law also attempted to encourage efforts to prevent human trafficking internationally, by creating annual country reports on trafficking, as well as by tying financial non-humanitarian assistance to foreign countries to real efforts in addressing human trafficking.

International NPOs, such as Human Rights Watch and Amnesty International, have called on the United States to improve its measures aimed at reducing trafficking. They recommend that the United States more fully implement the "United Nations Protocol to Prevent, Suppress and Punish Trafficking in Persons, Especially Women and Children" and the "United Nations Convention against Transnational Organized Crime" and for immigration officers to improve their awareness of trafficking and support the victims of trafficking.

United States State Law on Trafficking Several states have also written laws to address human trafficking in their borders. Florida has written trafficking statutes criminalizing forced labor, sex trafficking, and document servitude. Florida also provides for mandatory law enforcement trainings and victim services.

On May 8, 2006, Connecticut passed an act addressing human trafficking that criminalized coerced work, and made trafficking a violation of the Connecticut RICO Act.

Human Trafficking in Popular Culture

Lilya 4-ever, a film based loosely on the real life of Dangoule Rasalaite, portrays a young woman from the former Soviet Union who is deceived into being trafficked for exploitation in Sweden. Human trafficking has also been portrayed in the Canadian/UK TV drama Sex Traffic. Based on true events, Svetlana's Journey by Michael Cory Davis depicts the trials of a 13-year-old who loses her family and is sold to human traffickers by her adoptive family. Drugged, raped, and forced to endure continuous abuse by her 'clients' and traffickers, she finally commits suicide. The 2007 film Trade deals with human trafficking out of Mexico and a brother's attempt to rescue his kidnapped and trafficked young sister. It is based on Peter Landesman's article about sex slaves, which was featured as the cover story in the January 24, 2004 issue of New York Times Magazine.

The film The Transporter deals with the hero, Frank Martin, played by Jason Statham, trying to stop a container full of men and women being illegally transported. Human Trafficking (2005) (TV) by Christian Duguay stars Mira Sorvino, Donald Sutherland, and Richard Carlyle. A sixteen-year-old girl from the Ukraine, a single mother from Russia, an orphaned seventeen-year-old girl from Romania, and a twelve-year-old American tourist become the victims of international sex slave traffickers. Sorvino and Sutherland are the Immigration and Customs Enforcement (ICE) agents who struggle to save them.

FREE INDEPENDENT TRAVELER/TOURIST (FIT)

With world travel market having undergone significant changes over the last few years a new type of tourist has emerged known as the Free Independent Traveler or Tourist (FIT). The definition is broad but tends to refer to people over 35, often, though not necessarily, of above average income who like to travel in small groups, usually couples. They eschew mass tourism and the holiday package concept promoted by Travel operators, in favour of a more individualistic approach to travel. There are two implications to the idea of the Free Independent Traveler. One is important in the context of a marketing niche with a distinct economic behaviour whilst the other concentrates more on the philosophy of travel. This distinction can be summarised in how they are described. For the economic importance of tourism and for marketing purposes they are Free Independent Travelers (Upper case as they are an identifiable group within the market) whilst the people themselves are perhaps more attracted to the possibilities and lack of limitations in the concept of being a free, independent traveler.

Free Independent Travelers as an Alternative Movement

They tend to be environmentally aware, enjoy experiencing new ways of life and are enthusiastic, off the beaten track explorers practising for travel what the Slow Food Movement does for eating. They enjoy good food, architecture, and the heritage of local cultures. They tend to reject the traditional Package holiday model and even the Dynamic packaging system of doing things. People may garner information from a wide variety of sources or tips. The Guardian Newspaper's ivebeenthere site or Lonely Planet's forum are all examples and represent the fundamental difference between the FIT and other types of travel that this is about sharing and passing on of ideas and knowledge in accordance with the much talked about Web 2.0. The FIT vacation is a custom built cocktail then with suggestions from friends, forums, speciality providers or others creating the idea around which the vacation is built. The FITs themselves are responsible for adding components in place of the traditional package operators. The rise of low cost airlines in the US and Europe has also increased the supply of alternative and lower cost short haul destinations fueling demand for these newly available markets. Southwest Airlines in the US, Ryanair and easyJet in Europe and later Spanish, German and nationally orientated airlines grew up adding destinations and creating an internationally networked portfolio of air-routes delivering people to destinations that were not previously available at a commercial, international level.

The internet is fundamental to the rise of the FIT, offering them the suggestions, for example, of a good meal out in Rome from a fellow FIT, across the globe, who ate there last week.

Free Independent Travelers as an Economic Phenomenon

Here they are an important and growing sector in the market. Governments, regional tourist boards and other public sectors responsible for tourism development try to attract them. Why? The basic principle is economics. FITs spread their money around in a more efficient fashion. Fifteen FITs will eat, sleep, snack, take a coffee, go to theatres/art shows/opera festivals/ football games/rural villages in fifteen different locations and introduce their money in hundreds of different channels harnessing the power of Keynes' multiplier effect in a much more efficient manner.

Contrast this with a group tour of another 15 people run by Tour Operator 1 based in and delivering share-holder profit to Country A. Their tour to Country B is less efficient from an economic development point of view as the Tour Operator controls so many of the components in the chain. Also those 15 sleep in the same hotel and eat in the same restaurants ensuring that though their money stimulates the local economy it tends to do so in a less than optimally efficient manner.

GARDEN TOURISM

Garden tourism is a type of niche tourism involving visits or travel to botanical gardens and places which are significant in the history of gardening. Garden tourists often travel individually in countries with which they are familiar but often prefer to join organized garden tours in countries where they might experience difficulties with language, travel or finding accommodation in the vicinity of the garden.

The list of famous gardens which attract garden tourists from afar includes: Sissinghurst Castle Garden and Stourhead in England, Versailles and Giverny in France, Keukenhof in Holland, Villa d'Este and Villa Lante in Italy, Alhambra in Spain, Longwood Gardens and Filoli in the USA, Taj Mahal in India, Ryoan-ji in Japan. In the year 2000 the Alhambra and the Taj Mahal both received over 2 million visitors. This poses problems for the landscape manager.

Michel de Montaigne was one of the earliest garden tourists to record his impressions of gardens (c1580). John Evelyn also recorded his visits to gardens in France and Italy, as did Fynes Moryson. At the start of the twenty-first century Britain had the largest number of gardens open to the public for tourist visits: over 3,500 gardens are listed in Gardens of England and Wales Open for Charity (the 'Yellow Book').

GUEST RANCH

The guest ranch, also known as a dude ranch, is a type of ranch oriented towards visitors or tourism. It is a phenomenon of the romanticization of the American West after the official closing of the United States frontier in the late 19th century. The Western adventures of hardy aristocrats like Theodore Roosevelt were made available to paying guests from cities or the East, called "tenderfeet," "greenhorns," or "dudes" in the West. After World War I, the transcontinental railroad network brought these paying visitors to the local depot, where a wagon would be waiting for them. Some guest ranch visitors expected a somewhat edited version of the "cowboy life," while others were more tolerant of the odors and timetable of a working ranch. Guest ranches have also become a feature of the Australian Outback.

In the United States, guest ranches are a long-established tradition and continue to be a popular vacation destination. Depending on the climate, some guest ranches are open only in the summer or winter, others offer "year-round" service in all four seasons. College students are often recruited to work at guest ranches during the summer months. Common jobs offered to college students include: housekeeping, wrangler, dining staff, and office staff or babysitters.

Hunting Ranches

Some guest ranches cater to hunters. Some feature native wildlife such as whitetail deer, mule deer, bison or elk. Others feature exotic species imported from other nations such as Africa and India. Both types of ranches are highly controversial. While many traditional ranches allow hunters and outfitters on their land to hunt native game, the act of confining game to guarantee a kill is considered unsporting by some people.

The introduction of non-native species on ranches is even more controversial because of concerns that these "exotics" may escape and contaminate the gene pool of native species or spread previously unknown disease. The advocates of hunting ranches argue in turn that they help protect native herds from over-hunting and the stocking of exotic species actually increases their numbers and may help save them from extinction.

HERITAGE TOURISM

Cultural heritage tourism (or just heritage tourism) is a branch of tourism oriented towards the cultural heritage of the location where tourism is occurring. Culture has always been a major object of travel, as the development of the Grand Tour from the 16th century onwards attests. In the 20th century, some people have claimed, culture ceased to be the objective of tourism: tourism is now culture. Cultural attractions play an important role in tourism at all levels, from the global highlights of world culture to attractions that underpin local identities. (Richards, 1996)

According to the Weiler and Hall, culture, heritage and the arts have long contributed to appeal of tourist destination. However, in recent years 'culture' has been rediscovered as an important marketing tool to attract those travellers with special interests in heritage and arts. According to the Hollinshead, cultural heritage tourism defines as cultural heritage tourism is the fastest growing segment of the tourism industry because there is a trend toward an increase specialization among tourist. This trend is evident in the rise in the volume of tourists who seek adventure, culture, history, archaeology and interaction with local people.

Cultural heritage tourism is important for various reasons; it has a positive economic and social impact, it establishes and reinforces identity, it helps preserve the cultural heritage, with culture as an instrument it facilitates harmony and under-standing among people, it supports culture and helps renew tourism (Richards, 1996).

Cultural heritage tourism has a number of objectives that must be met within the context of sustainable development such as; the conservation of cultural resources, accurate interpretation of resources, authentic visitors experience, and the stimulation of the earned revenues of cultural resources. We can see therefore, that cultural heritage tourism is not only concerned with identification, management and protection of the heritage values but it must also be involved in understanding the impact of tourism on communities and regions, achieving economic and social benefits, providing financial resources for protection, as well as marketing and promotion. (J. M. Fladmark, 1994)

Heritage tourism involves visiting historical or industrial sites that may include old canals, railways, battlegrounds, etc. The overall purpose is to gain an appreciation of the past. It also refers to the marketing of a location to members of a diaspora who have distant family roots there. Decolonization and immigration form the major background of much contemporary heritage tourism. Falling travel costs have also made heritage tourism possible for more people.

Another possible form involves religious travel or pilgrimages. Many Catholics from around the world come to the Vatican and other sites such as Lourdes or Fátima. Large numbers of Jews have both visited Israel and emigrated there. Many have also gone to Holocaust sites and memorials. Islam commands its followers to take the hajj to Mecca, thus differentiating it somewhat from tourism in the usual sense, though the trip can also be a culturally important event for the pilgrim. Heritage Tourism can also be attributed to historical events that have been dramatised to make them more entertaining. For example a historical tour of a town or city using a theme such as ghosts or vikings.

LITERARY TOURISM

Literary Tourism is a type of cultural tourism that deals with places and events from fictional texts as well as the lives of their authors. This could include following the route a fictional character charts in a novel, visiting particular settings from a story or tracking down the haunts of a novelist. Literary tourists are specifically interested in how places have influenced writing and at the same time how writing has created place. In order to become a literary tourist you only need a novel and an inquisitive mind-set, however there are literary guides, literary maps and literary tours to help you on your way. In addition to visiting author and book sites, literary tourists often engage in bookstore tourism, browsing local bookshops for titles specifically related to the sites as well as other regional books and authors.

Literary Tourism in KwaZulu-Natal

'Literary Tourism in KwaZulu-Natal' is a National Research Foundation funded project that is working on a Literary Map that connects authors whose lives or work is tied in some significant way to specific places in KwaZulu-Natal, South Africa. Each author entry contains a short biography, a selected bibliography and an excerpt from the author's work that relates to the place identified in the map. The map can be viewed here:

MUSIC TOURISM

Music tourism is the act of visiting a city or town in order to see a gig or festival. With the presence of the tourist, money is spent and the local economy benefits. This sort of tourism is particularly important to small villages such as Glastonbury, as well as large cities like Glasgow.

NAKED HIKING

Naked walking, naked hiking, or Freehiking is a sub-set of the modern form of social nudity. For some people, naked hiking may appear to be some form of energetic sport; however, for most it is simply a pleasant recreational pastime, with no social agenda.

Context

Naturism has traditionally been an activity engaged in a private space or landed club environment. Modern naturism is moving towards a public space, as well including a more active component. Although naturists have always been interested in health and fitness, indeed this was a prerequisite to many early gatherings, and most clubs have volleyball nets and table tennis tables, there has always been a slight reluctance to walk, run or cycle naked. One reason for this has been the secluded nature of the early clubs, private from prying eyes and textiles, and the limited area in which the early pioneers had to work with.

Modern naturism in nude-tolerant societies is moving out of the private enclosure and towards the arena of public nudity, where it is deemed ok to be not only naked in public, but where it is also ok to be active (from a stroll to action sports) in the nude. The point about being active is that many people appear to find static nudity acceptable, for example in the media (porn magazines or page 3 girls in newspapers), and theatre (non-moving Greek-statue-like nudity), but moving nudity, in contrast, seems to generate heated feeling.

Attention and Opinion

Naked outdoor activity is a subject expounded clearly in the publications of the Nacktiv site. People simply go about their normal day to day business, or recreational activities, naked. The more naked bodies people see in a public setting the more likely they are to question the advertising and media industries' onesided linking of sex with nudity. Public active nudists go out of their way to be discreet, and are to be seen walking in remote mountain areas, through quiet forests and woods, across distant fields and scrubland, and not in densely populated areas, often not meeting anyone else at all. In the United Kingdom, Steve Gough, known as The Naked Rambler, received much media coverage for walking naked from Land's End to John o' Groats in 2003-2004 and again in 2005-2006. He was arrested and imprisoned several times during both his walks. In both 2005 and 2006 the European Alps were crossed naked during a one week hiking (tour), there was little media coverage and no-one was arrested or troubled.

Special Considerations

Although extremists might insist that naked hiking should be all-naked, and nothing but naked, as in all things one should remain practical and sensible about such activities.

Sensible footwear might mean bare feet on the beach, but wearing mountain boots in the mountains. Sunstroke or sunburn is a danger by any activity, naked or not, but naked hiking in the high mountains exposes the body to an increased level of sunshine not found at sea level, so sunscreen and a sun hat are essential items. Bugs, such as mosquitoes and midges, can be particularly troublesome, especially in sensitive areas, so anti-bug formulas are often needed by participants in this activity. Walking through a bunch of stinging nettles, or a field full of high thistles, can be an interesting experience (even with shorts on). Naturally, extra care must be taken.

NEO TOURISM

Neo Tourism is a term coined by the Korea tourism organization that comprehensively describes the newly changing trend of the tourism.

Definition of Neo Tourism

Following the changes in the economic, social and cultural paradigm of the last century, the form of tourism is changing as well. "Neo Tourism" is a term that comprehensively describes the new aspects of such changes and diversification of the tourism. The "Neo Tourism" incorporates concepts such as 'Sustainable tourism' which puts emphasis on the environmental sustainability and 'Special Interest Tourism (SIT)' which reflects postmodern social phenomenon.

The Origin of Neo Tourism

Initially the term "Neo Tourism" was generated to explain a form of tourism which has not existed before, to say, "New Tourism". However, with continuous advents of various types of tourism, it has become necessary to categorize those concepts in further details and eventually the "Neo Tourism" has taken more concrete meaning as such including the essential key words in the category. Those essential key words are as follows.

- Postmodernism
- Sustainability
- Digitalization

Application of Neo Tourism

The term of "Neo Tourism" can explain the following types of tourism.

- Tourism that satisfies individual interests and purposes appearing with post-modern social change

- Tourism that avoids the environmental destruction and ensure experiencing the untouched nature
- Tourism that manages various matters such as gathering information and making reservation through Internet.

The term "Neo Tourism" can be used from the suppliers' point of view as well as the customers' in the following concepts.

- Creating a new type of tourism product by connecting tourism industry with other industries. (ex. Medical tourism, Edu Tourism)
- Developing environmentally and socially sustainable tourist attractions
- Utilizing IT technology such as internet and ubiquitous systems to promote and sale the tourism products

POP-CULTURE TOURISM

Pop-culture tourism is the act of traveling to locations featured in literature, film, music, or any other form of popular entertainment.

Popular destinations have included:

- Los Angeles, California film studios.
- the Iowa cornfields featured in Field of Dreams
- New Zealand after The Lord of the Rings was filmed there
- The Louvre in which the book and movie The Da Vinci Code takes place
- Tom's Restaurant which is known to many as Monk's from Seinfeld
- Prince Edward Island, in which the Canadian novel Anne of Green Gables takes place, is a popular attraction for tourists, notably from Japan.
- South Korea because of the recent Hallyu phenomenon in East Asia.
- Japan for japanophiles or lovers of Japanese pop-culture.

- North Bend, Washington and in particular Twede's Cafe where much of the television show Twin Peaks was shot.
- Roslyn, Washington, which stood in for Cicely Alaska in the television show Northern Exposure.
- Tunisia, location of the filming of the Star Wars movies.

Pop-culture tourism is in some respects akin to pilgrimage, with its modern equivalents of places of pilgrimage, such as Elvis Presley's Graceland and the grave of Jim Morrison in Père Lachaise Cemetery. Another pop-culture tourism destination is Vulcan, Alberta Canada. In the early 1990s this small rural community began to explore ways it could capitalize on the coincidence of the Town's name being the same as popular Star Trek Character, Mr. Spock's home planet: Vulcan, to develop its local tourism industry.

PERPETUAL TRAVELER

The term perpetual traveler (PT, permanent tourist or prior taxpayer) refers to both a lifestyle and a philosophy.

Background

In practical terms, perpetual travelers are people who live in such a way that they are not considered a legal resident of any of the countries in which they spend time. In this way, they seek to avoid the legal obligations which may accompany residency, such as taxes, jury duty, and military service. For example, while PT's may hold citizenship in one or more countries that impose taxes based solely on residency, their legal residence will most likely be in a tax haven. They may spend the majority of their time in other countries, never staying long enough to be considered a resident.

Tax Avoidance

It is possible to live for several months, and in some cases even own property, in many countries without paying income tax. For example, one can spend up to 122 days each year in the United States without being considered a resident or being required to file a US tax return.

Some PT's are wealthy individuals whose primary motivation is tax avoidance. By exploiting the rules in place for tourists and travelers, individuals may be able to legally reduce or eliminate their tax burden. However other PT's, such as itinerants, may adopt this lifestyle for purely self-ownership reasons, just to be free from government authority, interference and "The System".

Five Flag Theory

Many perpetual travelers attempt to organize their affairs around the "Five Flags" theory, arranging for different facets of their lives to fall under the jurisdiction of separate countries, or flags. This is an extension of W.G. Hill's original "Three Flags" approach. Whether to minimize governmental interference (via taxes or otherwise), or to maximize privacy, the theory proposes that you arrange for each of the following to be in a separate country:

1. Passport and Citizenship-in a country that does not tax money earned outside the country
2. Legal Residence-in a tax haven
3. Business Base-where you earn your money
4. Asset Haven-where you keep your money
5. Playgrounds-where you spend your money

Philosophy

On the surface, perpetual tourists have some things in common with world citizens, in that they see themselves as untethered to any one nation. However, PT's generally seem to eschew the humanistic and utopian overtones of world citizenship. Many PT's align themselves closely with the libertarian school of thought, which advocates individual sovereignty-sovereignty vested in the individual rather than in nation-states.

PILGRIMAGE

In religion and spirituality, a pilgrimage is a long journey or search of great moral significance. Sometimes, it is a journey to a sacred place or shrine of importance to a person's beliefs and faith. Members of every major religion participate in pilgrimages. A person who makes such a journey is called a pilgrim.

Buddhism offers four sites of pilgrimage: the Buddha's birthplace at Kapilavastu, the site where he attained Enlightenment Bodh Gaya, where he first preached at Benares, and where he achieved Parinirvana at Kusinagara.

In the kingdoms of Israel and Judah the visitation of certain ancient cult-centers was repressed in the 7th century BC, when the worship was restricted to Jahweh at the temple in Jerusalem. In Syria, the shrine of Astarte at the headwater spring of the river Adonis survived until it was destroyed by order of Emperor Constantine in the 4th century AD.

In mainland Greece, a stream of individuals made their way to Delphi or the oracle of Zeus at Dodona, and once every four years, at the period of the Olympic games, the temple of Zeus at Olympia formed the goal of swarms of pilgrims from every part of the Hellenic world.

When Alexander the Great reached Egypt, he put his whole vast enterprise on hold, while he made his way with a small band deep into the Libyan desert, to consult the oracle of Ammun. During the imperium of his Ptolemaic heirs, the shrine of Isis at Philae received many votive inscriptions from Greeks on behalf of their kindred far away at home.

Although a pilgrimage is normally viewed in the context of religion, the personality cults cultivated by communist leaders ironically gave birth to pilgrimages of their own. Prior to the demise of the USSR in 1991, a visit to Lenin's Mausoleum in Red Square, Moscow can be said to have had all the characteristics exhibiting a pilgrimage-for Communists. This type of pilgrimage to a personality cult is still evident today on people who pay visits of homage to Mao Tse Tung, Kim Il Sung, and Ho Chi Minh.

Effects on Trade

Pilgrims contributed an important element to long-distance trade before the modern era, and brought prosperity to successful pilgrimage sites, an economic phenomenon unequalled until the tourist trade of the 20th century. Encouraging pilgrims was a motivation for assembling (and sometimes fabricating) relics and for writing hagiographies of local saints, filled with inspiring accounts of miracle cures. Lourdes and other modern pilgrimage sites keep this spirit alive.

Modern Pilgrimage

Pilgrimages are still made throughout the world: modern-day pilgrimages include the Way of St. James, the Hajj, and the pilgrimage to Mount Kailash. In modern usage, the terms pilgrim and pilgrimage can also have a somewhat devalued meaning as they are often applied in a secular context. For example, fans of Elvis Presley may choose to visit his home, Graceland, in Memphis, Tennessee. Similarly one may refer to a cultural center such as Venice as a "tourists' Mecca".

PILGRIMAGE CENTRES IN VARIOUS TIMES AND CULTURES

Antiquity

Many ancient religions had holy sites, temples and groves, where pilgrimages were made.

- Karnak, Egypt.
- Thebes, Egypt.
- Kurukshetra, India
- Delphi, Greece. Oracle.
- Dodona, Epirus, Greece. Oracle.
- Ephesus Temple of Diana.
- Baalbek Lebanon.

Bahá'í Faith

A Bahá'í pilgrimage currently consists of visiting the holy places in Haifa, Akká, and Bahjí in Northwest Israel. Bahá'ís do not have access to other places designated as sites for pilgrimage.

Bahá'u'lláh decreed pilgrimage in His Motherbook (Kitáb-i-Aqdas) to two places: the House of Bahá'u'lláh in Baghdad, Iraq, and the House of the Báb in Shiraz, Iran. In two separate Tablets, known as Suriy-i-Hajj, He prescribed specific rites for each of these pilgrimages (lifting the injunction regarding the shaving of one's head for pilgrimage in the Kitáb-i-Aqdas). It is obligatory to make the pilgrimage, "if one can afford it and is able to do so, and if no obstacle stands in one's way". Bahá'ís are free to choose between the two Houses, as either has been deemed sufficient. And although women are not bound to perform pilgrimage, they are certainly not prohibited to do so.

Later, 'Abdu'l-Bahá designated the Shrine of Bahá'u'lláh at Bahji (the Qiblih) as a site of visitation. No rites have been prescribed for this.

Buddhism

Gautama Buddha spoke of the four sites most worthy of pilgrimage for his followers to visit:

- Lumbini: birth place (in Nepal)
- Bodh Gaya: place of Enlightenment
- Sarnath: (formally Isipathana) where he delivered his first teaching
- Kusinara: (now Kusinagar, India) where he attained mahaparinirvana (passed away).

Other pilgrimage places in India and Nepal connected to the life of Gautama Buddha are: Savatthi, Pataliputta, Nalanda, Gaya, Vesali, Sankasia, Kapilavastu, Kosambi, Rajagaha, Varanasi.

Other famous places for buddhist pilgrimage in various countries include:

- India: Sanchi, Ellora, Ajanta.
- Thailand: Sukhothai, Ayutthaya, Wat Phra Kaew, Wat Doi Suthep.
- Tibet: Lhasa (traditional home of the Dalai Lama), Mount Kailash, Lake Nam-tso.

- Cambodia: Angkor Wat, Silver Pagoda.
- Sri Lanka: Polonnaruwa, Temple of the Tooth (Kandy), Anuradhapura.
- Laos: Luang Prabang.
- Myanmar: Bagan, Sagaing Hill.
- Nepal: Bodhnath, Swayambhunath.
- Indonesia: Borobudur.
- China: Yung-kang, Lung-men caves.
- Japan: Kyoto, Nara.

Communism

- USSR: Moscow, Mausoleum of Lenin in Red Square.
- China: Peking, Mausoleum of Mao Tse Tung in Tiananmen Square.
- Germany: Trier, Birthplace of Karl Marx in Trier

Christianity

Pilgrimages were first made to sites connected with the birth, life, crucifixion and resurrection of Jesus. Surviving descriptions of Christian pilgrimages to the Holy Land date from the 4th century, when pilgrimage was encouraged by church fathers like Saint Jerome. Pilgrimages also began to be made to Rome and other sites associated with the Apostles, Saints and Christian martyrs, as well as to places where there have been apparitions of the Virgin Mary. The crusades to the holy land are also considered to be mass armed pilgrimages.

The second largest single pilgrimage in the history of Christendom was to the Funeral of Pope John Paul II after his death on April 2, 2005. An estimated four million people travelled to Vatican City, in addition to the almost three million people already living in Rome, to see the body of Pope John Paul II lie in state.

World Youth Day is a major Catholic Pilgrimage, specifically for people aged 16-35. It is held internationally every 2-3 years. In 2005, young Catholics visited Cologne, Germany. In

1995, the largest gathering of all time was to World Youth Day in Manila, Philippines, where four million people from all over the world attended. The major Christian pilgrimages are to:

- Jerusalem. Site of the crucifixion and resurrection of Jesus.
- Rome on roads such as the Via Francigena. Site of the deaths of Saint Peter, Saint Paul and other early martyrs. Location of sacred relics of various saints, relics of the Passion, important churches and headquarters of the Catholic Church.
- Constantinople (today Istanbul, Turkey). Former capital of the Byzantine Empire and the see of one of the five ancient Patriarchates and spiritual see of the Eastern Orthodox Church. Hagia Sophia, former cathedral and burial place of many Ecumenical Patriarchs.
- Lourdes, France. Apparition of the Virgin Mary. The second most visited Christian pilgrimage site after Rome.
- Santiago de Compostela in Spain on the Way of St James (Spanish: El Camino de Santiago). This famous medieval pilgrimage to the shrine of Saint James is still popular today.

Other important Christian pilgrimage sites include:

- Assisi, Italy, St. Francis of Assisi and St Clare, relics
- Ávila, Spain, St Theresa of Avila, relics
- Bethlehem, in Israel, Birthplace of Jesus and King David.
- Canterbury Cathedral associated with Saint Thomas Becket.
- Cap-de-la-Madeleine, Quebec, Canada in honour of Our Lady of the Cape.
- Cathedral of Chartres, France.
- Miercurea Ciuc, Transylvania, Romania. Whit Sunday gathering of (mostly ethnic Hungarian) Catholics.

- Croagh Patrick, Ireland. Saint Patrick.
- Conques, France
- Cologne, Germany. Relics of the Three Magi.
- Czestochowa, Poland.Black Madonna of Czestochowa is housed pernamently in theJasna Góra Monastery
- Glastonbury, England. St Joseph of Arimathea.
- Goa, India. St. Francis Xavier
- Hill of Crosses, Lithuania
- House of the Virgin Mary, Turkey. Pope John-Paul II declared the Shrine of Virgin Mary as a pilgrimage place for Christians.
- Issoudun, France. Notre-Dame du Sacré-Coeur
- Kapel in 't Zand, Limburg
- Kevelaer, Germany
- Knock, Ireland
- Lichen, Sanctuary of Our Lady of Lichen
- Lisieux, France. Saint Therese of Lisieux, burial place.
- Lourdes, France. Apparition of the Virgin Mary. Place of healing.
- Mariazell, Austria. Marian Shrine to Austria and Hungary
- Medugorje, Bosnia-Herzegovina. Apparitions of the Virgin Mary at the present.
- Mount Athos, Greece. Orthodox monastic centre.
- Mount Nebo, Jordan. Traditional site of the death of Moses.
- Mount Sinai, Egypt, holy mountain to the ancient Hebrews, traditional site has been commemorated since time of Constantine
- Nazareth, Israel, hometown of Jesus
- Fatima, Portugal. Apparition of the Virgin Mary.

- Padua, Italy, St Anthony, relics
- Paris (Sacred-Heart Basilica Basilica of the Sacré Cœur; and Saint Catherine Labouré)
- Rosslyn Chapel, Scotland
- Sacri Monti, Italy. The Sacred Mountains of Piedmont and Lombardy.
- San Giovanni Rotondo, Italy, St Pio from Pietrelcina
- Guadalupe, Spain
- Sea of Galilee, Israel, site of Jesus' early ministry.
- Shrine of Our Lady of Guadalupe, Mexico City. Apparition of the Virgin Mary.
- St. Andrews, Scotland, it is said that Saint Andrew was given, by God, directions to the location of St Andrews
- St. Patrick's Purgatory, Donegal, Ireland
- St. Thomas Mount, India. Place where St. Thomas was martyed.
- Taizé Community, France, modern monastery that actively encourages pilgrimages to it
- Nidaros Cathedral, Norway
- Turin, Italy. Holy Shroud.
- Vailankanni, India. 16th-century Mary apparition site.
- Vierzehnheiligen, Germany.
- Walsingham, England. Virgin Mary apparition site.
- Wittenberg, Germany. Church of Martin Luther and centre of the Protestant Reformation.

Hinduism

Hindus are required to undertake pilgrimages during their lifetime. Most Hindus who can afford to go on such journeys travel to numerous sites including those below:

- Badrinath
- Kedarnath

- Gangotri
- Yamunotri
- Rishikesh
- Haridwar
- Benares
- Mandher Devi temple in Mandhradevi
- Vrindavan
- Mayapur
- Udupi
- Kateel
- Talapady
- Tirupati
- Palani
- Kukke Subramanya

The first four sites in the list above together comprise the Chardham, or four holy pilgrimage destinations. It is believed that travelling to these places leads to moksha, the release from samsara (cycle of rebirths).

Vrindavan is most important place of pilgrimage for every Vaishnava, especially for the followers of Gaudiya Vaishnavism who regard Krishna as the original Personality of Godhead (God). Here one can attain love of God (prema).

Islam

Pilgrimage to Mecca-the Hajj-is one of the Five Pillars of Islam. It should be attempted at least once in the lifetime of all able-bodied Muslims who can afford to do so. It is the most important of all Muslim Pilgrimages.

Many Muslims also undergo ziyarat, which is a pilgrimage to sites associated with the prophet Muhammad, his companions, or other venerated figures in Islamic history, such as Shi'a imams or Sufi saints. Sites of pilgrimage include mosques, graves, battlefields, mountains, and caves. Local

Pilgrimage traditions-those undertaken as ziarah visits to local graves, are also found throughout Muslim countries. In some countries, the grave sites of heroes have very strong ziyarah traditions as visiting the graves at auspicious times is a display of national and community identity. Some traditions within Islam have negative attitudes towards grave visiting.

The third religiously sanctioned pilgrimage for Muslims is to the Al Quds mount in Jerusalem which hosts Al-Aqsa Mosque and the Dome of the Rock.

Judaism

Within Judaism, the Temple in Jerusalem was the center of the Jewish religion, until its destruction in 70 AD, and all who were able were under obligation to visit and offer sacrifices known as the korbanot, particularly during the Jewish holidays in Jerusalem.

Following the destruction of the Second Temple and the onset of the diaspora, the centrality of pilgrimage to Jerusalem in Judaism was discontinued.

In its place came prayers and rituals hoping for a return to Zion and the accompanying restoration of regular pilgrimages (see Jerusalem, Jews and Judaism).

Until recent centuries, pilgrimage has been a fairly difficult and arduous adventure. But now, Jews from many countries make periodic pilgrimages to the holy sites of their religion.

The western retaining wall of the original temple, known as the Wailing Wall, or Western Wall remains in the Old City of Jerusalem and this has been the most sacred site for Zionist Jews.

Pilgrimage to this area was off-limits from 1948 to 1967, when East Jerusalem was controlled by Jordan. Some Reform and Conservative Jews who no longer consider themselves exiles, still enjoy visiting Israel even if it is not an official "pilgrimage."

SACRED TRAVEL

Sacred travel, or metaphysical tourism, is a growing niche of the travel market. It attracts New Age believers, primarily middle-aged women, and involves tours and travel to "spiritual hotspots" on the Earth.

Destinations are often ancient sites where there is a mystery concerning their origin or purpose, such as Machu Picchu in Peru, The Pyramids of Egypt, or Stonehenge in England. Some Christian sites such as the locations of the Black Madonnas and the Rosslyn Chapel in Scotland are also popular.

These travelers see the journey as more than just tourism and take the trips in order to heal themselves and the world. Part of this may involve rituals involving, (supposedly), leaving their bodies, possession by spirits (channelling), and recovery of past life memories.

SAFARI

A safari is an overland journey. It usually refers to a trip by tourists to Africa, traditionally for a big-game hunt and in more modern times to watch and photograph big game and other wildlife as a safari holiday.

There is a certain theme or style associated with the word, which includes khaki clothing, pith helmets, and animal skins-like leopard's skin.

Etymology

Entering the English language in the late 19th century, the word safari means 'journey' in Swahili language. Originally from the Arabic (safara) meaning travel The verb for "to travel" in Swahili is "safiri", the noun for the journey is "safari". These words are used for any type of journey e.g. by bus from Nairobi to Mombasa.

Touristic Usage

Most people in the West still believe that a true safari can only be in East Africa, that is Kenya and Tanzania, and not in Africa as a whole.

That is to say that if you were in South Africa doing some big game watching, you wouldn't be "on safari" even though the word is broadly used, because the word "safari" comes from the Swahili-speaking people who can be found along the Swahili Coast. Today the word is used generally to mean anything from big game viewing, photography, or even game hunting.

VIRTUAL TOURISM

Virtual tourism refers to pre-planning alternative touristic activity before your departure, by integrating multiple digital resources to explore regions of the world without having to physically travel. It helps focus attention onto people, places and exploring changes over time.

By using the internet, travel literature (travel guides and travelogues), Journals, Papers and television visual learning courseware graphically shows information necessary to make an informed decision about which places to visit and historic or scenic byways to explore.

It is an economical activity that employs people from several different specific areas, such as journalists and photographers, geographers, editors, cameras, writers, etc... and it is one activity related to promoting nature-based or people-powered outdoor recreation involving adventure-based tourism.

VOLUNTEER VACATION

Volunteer vacations are an opportunity for people to make a positive difference in the lives of others or to help improve or contribute to society, culture, or the environment while on vacation.

It is also a chance for people of nearly any age to immerse themselves in foreign or challenging circumstances, experience a different culture first-hand, and learn more about the world they live in.

According to the Travel Industry Association of America, more than 55 million Americans have participated in a volunteer vacation, and about 100 million more are considering taking one. Volunteer vacations attract people from all walks of life and all age groups-students on break or who take a year off between high school and college, singles, couples, families with young children, and older adults.

Despite obvious differences among these people, they typically share a desire to "do something good" while also experiencing new places and challenges in locales they might not otherwise visit.

Choosing a Volunteer Vacation

People choose to take a volunteer vacation for a variety of reasons, and often more than one applies. First and foremost is a desire to help-be it children, the elderly, the handicapped, animals, or the natural environment.

Some people have a specific cause in mind; say, protecting endangered gorillas or preserving the coral reefs off the coast of Australia, and they target organizations that offer such opportunities. Other people have a more general idea of what they want to do; for example, help alleviate hunger or teach children to read.

Along with an altruistic reason for volunteering there are often others, such as a desire to see exotic or unusual places, an opportunity to experience new challenges, a chance to practice a foreign language, having an experience that will enhance their resume and/or job opportunities, and the fact that such trips usually provide a substantial tax deduction. When choosing a volunteer vacation opportunity, prospective travelers should consider several questions.

- Where to go?

  Volunteer vacation opportunities are available in every corner of the world, from the United States to Australia, China, Iceland, and the Amazon.

- How much does it cost?

  The program fees participants pay to take part in volunteer vacations typically (but not always) include room and board, project fees, travel medical insurance, and travel within the country in which the volunteer activity occurs. The fees usually do not include transportation to the country. Potential volunteers should check with the sponsoring organization to determine which costs are included in the program fee, and to learn how much of the fee is tax deductible.

- How challenging is it?

  Some volunteer vacations require a certain level of physical strength and stamina, especially those that involve working outdoors. Potential volunteers should always clearly understand the physical expectations and requirements and be sure they are medically capable of meeting them.

- What are the accommodations?

  Lodging options vary widely and may involve pitching a tent, living in unheated huts, staying with native families, sharing a dormitory-type residence, or checking into a comfortable hotel. Questions about food, water, linens, availability of power (including computer and cell phone access), medical care, and local transportation should be addressed during the evaluation process.

- How long?

  Most volunteer vacations last from one to four weeks; some can extend on for months. The vast variety of volunteer vacation opportunities usually means people can find more than one vacation that fits their needs.

- Any special skills needed?

  People who have special skills-teachers, nurses, veterinarians, biologists, accountants, lawyers, photographers, farmers-are always welcome and in fact urgently needed in some locations. Most volunteer opportunities, however, only ask that people have a desire to help and a willingness to learn and follow directions.

- Is language a barrier?

  Since so many volunteer vacations are in remote, foreign locations, knowledge of another language in addition to English can be helpful and in some cases, strongly recommended. However, most potential volunteers do not need to know a second language.

- What about free time?

  The amount of time volunteers have to spend sightseeing or doing other activities away from their volunteer tasks varies with each assignment, as do the types of activities that are available. This information is usually provided by the sponsoring organization, and it can be helpful to talk or correspond with other people who have volunteered in the location previously.

- Who can participate?

  Volunteer vacations are available for singles, couples, students, families, and older adults. The age limitation is typically 16 to 18 years of age; a parent or guardian usually must accompany any person younger than 16. Volunteer vacations geared for families with younger children have their own special regulations.

HOW TO FIND A VOLUNTEER VACATION

Both for-profit and nonprofit organizations and companies offer volunteer vacations. Some organizations sponsor opportunities that focus on a specific issue, such as saving sea turtles or building homes for the needy, while others offer a broad spectrum of projects that center on areas such as education, poverty, public health, endangered species, and habitat preservation.

While some organizations have projects in only a few countries, others offer options in dozens of locations on nearly every continent. People interested in learning more about volunteer vacations in general or selecting one in particular can begin by exploring volunteer vacation directories or targeting organizations that offer specific opportunities.

Volunteer Vacation Directories

People who are uncertain about the type of volunteer vacation they want to take may find it best to start by checking a directory of opportunities by category.

Charity Guide is a nonprofit that provides information on volunteer vacations in several different categories: environmental protection, children's issues, animal welfare, and health and safety. Travel with a Challenge provides a directory that caters to mature volunteers (age 45 years and older). Transitions Abroad is a portal for volunteer vacations involving social issues around the globe.

Organizations that Sponsor Volunteer Vacations

Potential volunteers can also scour the opportunities offered by organizations that sponsor volunteer vacations. Airline Ambassadors International distributes medical and other aid to children, families, and underprivileged communities around the world.

Global Service Corp. focuses its efforts in two countries, Tanzania and Thailand, and offers projects that last from two weeks up to six months.

People interested in environmental and animal issues can choose from more than 130 projects in 47 countries offered by the nonprofit group Earthwatch. Cross Cultural Solutions has projects lasting from one to twelve weeks located in eleven countries.

One-week opportunities are the mainstay of Globe Aware, which sponsors projects in nine countries. Community development, conservation, and teaching are just a few of the types of projects offered by i-to-i in more than two dozen countries. One unique type of organization is Peace Villages Foundation, a Non-Profit Franchise run and paid for entirely by volunteers.

People who don't find what they're looking for with a sponsoring organization or who have a pet cause or favorite charity can contact the particular group or charity on their own and ask about volunteer vacation opportunities.

WINE TOURISM

Wine tourism refers to tourism whose purpose is or includes the tasting, consumption, or purchase of wine, often at or near the source. Wine tourism can consist of visits to wineries, vineyards, and restaurants known to offer unique vintages, as well as organized wine tours, wine festivals, or other special events.

Many wine regions around the world have found it financially beneficial to promote such tourism; accordingly, growers associations and others in the hospitality industry in wine regions have spent significant amounts of money over the years to promote such tourism.

The National Wine Centre of Australia is a tourism venue that showcases the entire Australian wine industry. It is an education hub for tourists, the general public and full time students.

The National Wine Centre is a teaching centre for wine-related academic programs of The University of Adelaide, Australia. The University of Adelaide, "the wine university", is one of the top two educators in the world for wine studies along with the University of California-Davis.

SUSTAINABLE TOURISM

There are many different definitions of sustainable tourism, or responsible tourism, that have been developed over the last decade. Most tend to assume that all tourists are responsible for respecting and conserving a location's economic, environmental, and socio-cultural balances.

Global economists forecast continuing international tourism growth, ranging between three and six percent annually, depending on the location.

As one of the world's largest and fastest growing industries, this continuous growth will place great stress on remaining biodiverse habitats, often used to support mass tourism.

Sustainable tourists are aware of these dangers and seek to protect their favorite destinations, and to protect tourism as an industry. Sustainable tourists face many responsibilities to reduce tourism's impact on communities, including:

- informing themselves of the culture, politics, and economy of the communities being visited.
- anticipating and respecting local cultures' expectations and assumptions.
- contributing to intercultural understanding and tolerance.
- supporting the integrity of local cultures by favoring businesses which conserve cultural heritage
- supporting local economies by purchasing local goods and participating with small, local businesses.
- conserving resources by seeking out businesses that are environmentally conscious, and by using the least possible amount of non-renewable resources.

The Multilateral Investment Fund MIF Focus on destinations where there is already a critical mass of tourism businesses, MIF projects aim to boost the competitiveness of locally owned small and medium enterprises, helping them to organize themselves and work toward the shared goals of increasing income, employment and economic development.

See the Sustainable Tourism Action Plan and project proposal Guidelines.

Ecotourism

Ecotourism, according to Heather Robinson (2006), is a subset of sustainable tourism, differing by its focus on ecology.

Ecotourism is sustainable tourism that "contributes actively to the conservation of natural and cultural heritage; includes local and indigenous communities in its planning, development and operation, contributing to their well-being; interprets the natural and cultural heritage of the destination to visitors; and lends itself better to independent travellers, as well as to organized tours for small size groups.

In simple words ecotourism means while practicing any kind of tourism one should not harm nature.

For today's fast changing world only the practice of ecotourism can save nature from ever growing human population. Ecotourism is the best way to practice any kind of tourism whether it is wildlife tourism, adventure tourism, or heritage tourism.

It is the duty of all mankind to preserve nature and different species, only then can they survive for a long time; mankind should respect nature and its rules.

Man should preserve nature for the upcoming generation, so they also feel the pleasure of being in nature as people of this and earlier generations felt.

Bibliography

Apostolopulos, Y., S. Lewadi: The Sociology of Tourism, New York, Routledge, 1996.

Brogan, E.: Human Resource Development in Tourism: The Scottish Perspective, England, Wiley, 1994.

Cooper, C.: Tourism: Principles and Practice, London, Pitman, 1993.

Davies, I.: Competency Based Learning: Technology, Management, and Design, New York, McGraw-Hill, 1973.

Glenn Kreag, and John Sem: A Training Guide for Rural Tourism Development, Minnesota: Rural Tourism Center, 1995.

Gunn, Clare A.: Tourism Planning, New York, Crane Russak, 1979.

Hudman, Lloyd E.: Tourism: A Shrinking World, Columbus, Grid, 1980.

Ireland, Lewis: Quality Management for Projects and Programs, Upper Darby, PMI, 1991.

John Bowen, and James Makens: Marketing for Hospitality and Tourism: New Jersey, Prentice-Hall, 1998.

Knox, J.: Tourism Research Priorities in Hawaii and the Pacific, Honolulu, University of Hawaii, 1979.

Komilis, P.: Tourism and Sustainable Regional Development, Chichester, England, 1994.

Koth, Barbara: A Training Guide for Rural Tourism Development, Minnesota: Rural Tourism Center, 1995.

Kotler, Philip: Marketing for Hospitality and Tourism: New Jersey, Prentice-Hall, 1998.

Nelson, Bob and Economy, Peter: Managing for Dummies, Foster City, IDG Books, 1996.

Index

❑❑❑